WALKED OUT OF THE NEW ROAD

to

CONQUER CANCER

VOLUME II

Walked Out of the New Way of Cancer Treatment with Immune Regulation and Control of Combination of Chinese and Western Medicine

How to conquer cancer? How to treat cancer?

PART I

Authors: Xu Ze (China) ; Xu Jie(China) ; Bin Wu(America)
Translators: Bin Wu ; Lily Xu ; Zihao Xu ; Bo Wu
Editors: Bin Wu ; Lily Xu ; Tao Wu
Illustrators: Lily Xu ; Bin Wu

authorHOUSE®

AuthorHouse™
1663 Liberty Drive
Bloomington, IN 47403
www.authorhouse.com
Phone: 1 (800) 839-8640

AUTHORS: Xu Ze (China); Xu Jie(China); Bin Wu(America)
Translators: Bin Wu; Lily Xu; Zihao Xu; Bo Wu
Editors: Bin Wu; Lily Xu; Tao Wu
Illustrators: Lily Xu; Bin Wu

Published by AuthorHouse 01/25/2019

ISBN: 978-1-5462-7689-0 (sc)
ISBN: 978-1-5462-7745-3 (e)

Library of Congress Control Number: 2019900645

Print information available on the last page.

This book is printed on acid-free paper.

WALKED OUT OF THE NEW ROAD

to

CONQUER CANCER

New concepts or ideas of cancer treatment

Walked Out of the New Way of Cancer Treatment
with Immune Regulation and Control of Combination
of Chinese and Western Medicine

How to overcome cancer? How to treat cancer?

(Part I)

Contents

Foreword One

Foreword Two

First, the theoretical system of XZ-C immunomodulation and cancer treatment has been initially formed. Over the past 60 years, a new road to overcome cancer has been taken out. It is undergoing clinical application and observation verification.

Second, find the way

Third, the research on the new concept and new method of cancer metastasis

Introduction to this Book

Bin Wu

Science is endless and only those who are not afraid of danger or difficult work can reach the science peak. Dr. Xu Ze has been working in the cancer therapy for more than 60 years and works very hard day and night to do the basis and clinical oncology science for the patients and for our human being. In this book all of the contents are from his hard work and from his experiments and **from his excellent or superb surgery skills**, in which has two parts: Part I and Part II and three main topics are explained and demonstrated: 1. The reasons and the theoretical foundation of immune therapy, that is, **what is the theoretical basis of immune therapy which all of evidence are from his actual basic and clinical experiments; 2. How to use our immune therapy to treat the cancer patients? 3. Our clinical verification of our immune therapy is successful**. For example, During the animal experiments of making the tumor-bearing animal models, it was found that when Thymus was removed or the immune suppressor was used, the tumor-bearing animal models can be set up; **he found that immune function has close relation to cancer occurrence and metastasis.** During another of the cancer animal experiment, the body immune system can destroy 10^6 cancer cell so that the immune function should be protected and be activated and should be considered during the cancer prevention and treatment, etc, there are many new discoveries during the basic and clinical experiment. The most excellent things during his research are the series of anti-cancer and anti-cancer metastasis products or medications. After many years of difficult research and application of immune therapy together, the new road of cancer treatment have been working out. All of the contents in this book are the results and achievement of Dr. Xu Ze's hard work and his dedications to our human being and all of the contents are his talent scientific thinking and his high wisdom and his hard work day and night. Dr. Xu Ze has high surgery skills such as he made all of the tumor-bearing animal models and set up the animal modes for lymph and blood metastasis animal mode and the animal mode which the relations between hormone(pregnancy animal) and cancer, the animal model with cancer microcirculation and with the cancer new blood vessel formation which the new medications was found for stopping the tumor blood vessel growth, etc. **It needs the meticulous and high surgery skills to finish all of these procedure in the animal and in the human.** The dedication of Dr. Xu Ze is worth for all of us to learn. His oncology research model is based on **patient-centered** to discover question from clinical work, then come back to the in-depth animal experiments, and then turn to the clinical application in order to improve overall level of health care and ultimately the patient gets the benefits. **<u>The innovation brings the improvement and the progression.</u>**

Finally, due to finishing the books in such a short time and there are huge information in the book and day and night hard work, if there is any mistake, please forgive us and look forward to the feedback.

Bin Wu
12-18-2019 in Lutherville, Maryland in America

A Brief Introduction to The First Author

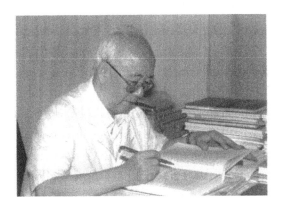

Xu Ze was born in 1933 in Leping City, Jiangxi Province in China. He graduated from Tongji Medical College in 1956. He served as the director of surgery, professor, chief physician, master and doctoral tutor of the Affiliated Hospital of Hubei College of Traditional Chinese Medicine. He is the director of the Experimental Surgery Research Institute of Hubei College of Traditional Chinese Medicine, director of the Department of Abdominal Oncology Surgery, and anti-cancer metastasis, the director of Recurrence Research Office; concurrently serves as executive director of Wuhan Branch of Chinese Medical Association, honorary president of Wuhan Anticancer Research Association, academic member of International Liver Disease Research Collaboration Center, member of International Federation of Surgeons, Chinese Journal of Experimental Surgery No. 1, 2, 3 The 4th Standing Editorial Board and the 1st, 2nd and 3rd Executive Editors of the Journal of Abdominal Surgery. He has been engaged in surgical work for 60 years and has extensive clinical experience in the surgical treatment of lung cancer, esophageal cancer, gastric cancer, liver cancer, gallbladder cancer, pancreatic cancer, and intestinal cancer etc, as well as the combination of Chinese and Western medicine to prevent postoperative recurrence and metastasis. In 1987, he began experimental research on tumors. Through cancer cell transplantation, he established tumor animal models, explored the mechanisms and rules of cancer metastasis and recurrence, and searched for ways to inhibit metastasis and screened 48 kinds of natural drugs from anti-cancer invasion and metastasis and relapsed Chinese medicine, and based on this, he developed xz-c immunomodulation anticancer traditional Chinese medicine preparation, which were clinically verified by a large number of cases and the effect is remarkable. He published 126 scientific research papers and published "New Understanding and New Model of Cancer Treatment", published by Hubei Science and Technology Publishing House and published by Xinhua Bookstore in 2001, In 2006, he published the monograph "New Concept and New Method of Cancer Metastasis Treatment" published by Beijing People's Military Medical Publishing House and published by Xinhua Bookstore. In April 2007, he was awarded the original book award and certificate by the General Administration of Press and Publication of the People's Republic of China. In October 2011, the third monograph (New Concepts and New Methods of Cancer Treatment) was published by Beijing People's Military Medical Press. Xu Ze, Xu Jie/ Zhang, Xinhua Bookstore was released. This book was translated into English by Dr. Bin Wu., published in Washington, DC on March 26, 2013, international distribution. He participated in 10 medical monographs such as "Hepatology Treatment" and "Abdominal Surgery". He engaged in teaching for 60 years, trained many young physicians, 10 master students And 2 doctoral students. He has been engaged in surgical research for 34 years and has achieved many results. Among them, "self-made XZ-C$_1$ type abdominal cavity-venous bypass device for the treatment of cirrhotic refractory ascites and its clinical application" was awarded the Hubei Provincial Government Science and Technology for the second prize of the results, and promoted and applied in 38 hospitals across the country: The National Natural Science Foundation of China's experimental study on the pathophysiology and pathogenesis of pulmonary schistosomiasis by experimental surgical methods won the second prize of Hubei Provincial Government Science and Technology Achievements. He enjoys Special government allowance.

A Brief Introduction to the Second Author

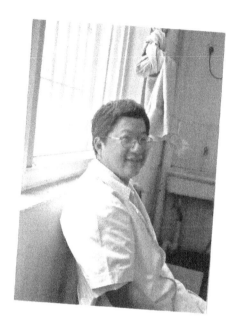

Xu Jie, male, graduated from Hubei College of Traditional Chinese Medicine in 1992, graduated from Hubei Medical University in 1996, Department of Clinical Medicine. Now He is chief physician in Hubei University of Traditional Chinese Medicine Hospital and Hubei Provincial Hospital of Surgery, engaged in experimental surgical tumor research and general surgery, urology clinical work.

Since 1992, he has been involved in the experimental tumor research of the Institute of Experimental Surgery of Hubei College of Traditional Chinese Medicine. He has carried out cancer cell transplantation and established a tumor animal model. He has carried out a series of experimental tumor research: exploring the mechanism of recurrence and metastasis of cancer and in vivo screening experiment of more than 200 kinds of Chinese herbal medicine in vivo tumor model of tumor inhibition s from a large number of natural medicine to find out, screening out of 48 kinds of anti-cancer invasion, metastasis, relapse traditional Chinese medicine

He participates in clinical validation and followed up for XZ - C immunoregulatory Chinese herbal medicine and completes the experimental research and clinical verification, data collection, collection and summary of this book.

A brief introduction to the third author and the main translator and the main editor

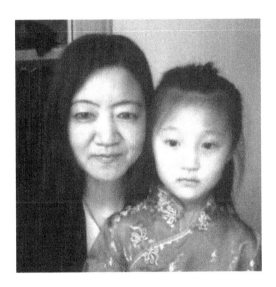

Bin Wu, MD, Ph.D., graduated from College of Yunyang of Tongji University of Medical Sciences for her MD degree; Studied her Master degree and her Ph. D degree in Sun Yat-Sen University of Medical Sciences. After she received her Ph.D., she worked as a Post-doctoral Follews in the Johns Hopkins Medical School and University of Maryland Medical School. She passed her USMLE tests and is going to do her residency training in America. She dedicated herself to oncology clinical and research. Her goal is to conquer cancer, which she believes this great contribution to our health. She has a daughter, named Lily Xu who drew all of the pictures in this book.

A Brief introduction to the illustrator and the advisor

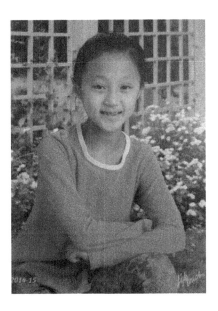

Lily Xu was born on November 17th 2006 and had an art presented in the Walter Art Museum in Baltimore at the age of 6; she got the fourth place trophy in the ES Double Digits or 24 and 24 games in the Baltimore County in Maryland; she got the first trophy in the BCPS STEM FAIR PHYSICS in Baltimore County; when she was in the sixth grade, she passed the advanced Math for 7th grade(which means the 8th grade math) test and moved the 8th grade math class; she loves the reading and the writing and she finished many series of books. She got $3000 scholarship award for the Peabody music program in the Johns Hopkins University. In 2018 she was chosen into Baltimore county Middle school Honor Band. In 2018 the robotic team which she attended for years got designing-award from the Baltimore county so that this robotic team will come to Maryland State for the Robotic contest. On January 19th, 2019 she got the Robotic designing- award in Maryland . She edits all of my books for the publishing and drew all of the pictures in this book.

Acknowledgements

This book is for all of people who concern human being health. We are deeply grateful to all of people who like our new ways to improve our human being health.

My daughter **Lily Xu** gave me many smart and creative ideas while we were finishing this book. Lily Xu drew all of the pictures such as the Thymus etc. **The characteristics of she loves the challenge** and **her judgment always encourages me to continue working hard to move on**.

I would like to express our sincere gratitude to the following:

1. All of Authorhouse staffs
2. Dr. Xu Ze's family and Dr. Xu Jie's family, especially his son Zihao Xu, who is the medical student in China
3. Mrs. Bo Wu's family and Mrs. Tao Wu's famly: espeicaly their daughters Chongshu Luo and Xunyue Wang

Bin Wu, M.D., Ph.D
12-18-2018 in Baltimore, Maryland in USA

I. The summary of the parts of our work and monography

Walked out of a new way of cancer treatment with the immune
regulation and control of the combination of Chinese and Western medicine

- Experimental *research: the study of Chinese medicine immunopharmacology and the combination of Chinese and Western medicine at the molecular level*
- *Walked out of a new path of cancer treatment with XZ-C immune regulation and control of the combination of Chinese and Western medicine at the molecular level*
- Walked *out a new way of conquering cancer with immune regulation and control, and regulating immune activity, and preventing thymus atrophy, and promoting thymic hyperplasia, and protecting bone marrow hematopoietic function, and improving immune surveillance, and combining Chinese medicine and Western medicine at the molecular level*
- The theoretical system of XZ-C immunoregulation *of cancer treatment and the theoretical basis and experimental basis of immunotherapy has been formed*
- We have embarked on the new road of cancer *treatment with XZ-C immune regulation and control, the combination of Chinese and Western medicine at the molecular level ----- "Chinese-style anti-cancer" new road*
- XZ-C immunomodulation anticancer Chinese medications are the result of the modernization of traditional Chinese medication.

(Part I)

Walked out of the new way of cancer treatment with immune
regulation and control of combination of Chinese and Western medicine

- Proposed or Presented a new finding in the experimental study of the etiology and pathogenesis of cancer in our laboratory: **"Thymus atrophy, low immune function is one of the causes and pathogenesis of cancer."**
- Due to the new findings of the above experimental research: **the principle of treatment** must be to prevent progressive atrophy of the thymus, promote thymic hyperplasia,

protect bone marrow hematopoietic function, improve immune surveillance, and control immune escape of malignant cells.

. **Provided the theoretical basis and experimental research basis of cancer immunotherapy with improving immune function.**

. As for at the cancer time, why does the thymus progressively shrink? XZ-C believes when the body has cancer, cancer cells may produce a cell inhibition factor that inhibits thymocyte proliferation. As for what is cytokine? We can call it "**cancer inhibiting thymus factor**" for the time being or temporarily. It is up to or waiting us to continue our experimental research. *(Part I)*

Under the guidance of Xi Jinping's new era of socialism with Chinese characteristics, we should strive to open up a new phase of scientific research in the new era, and the scientific research work to overcome cancer should be advanced. Strive to follow the path of independent innovation with Chinese characteristics and adhere to the road of independent innovation of Chinese and Western medicine combined with "Chinese-style anti-cancer". China will contribute more Chinese wisdom, China's programs, and China's power to the world, so that the sun of the humanity's destiny will shine in the world.

Walked out of the new road of cancer therapy with immune regulation and control of the combination of Chinese and western medicine

. Search or navigate a path or road
. Path finding and footprint
. Walking out of an XZ-C immune regulation and control of the combination of Chinese and Western medicine at the molecular level
. The theory system of cancer treatment of XZ-C immunoregulation has been formed, which is the theory basic and experimental basis of cancer immunotherapy
. A series products and adaptation range of XZ-C immune regulation and control anti-cancer Chinese medicine are provided or our research achievement
. XZ-C immunomodulation anticancer Chinese medicine is the result of the modernization of traditional Chinese medicine

How to overcome cancer? How to prevent cancer? How to treat cancer? How to overcome cancer and to launch the general attack of cancer?

Professor Xu Ze (XZ-C) summed up the collection, agglutinated wisdom, and proposed 1 to 8 of "walk out of a new path to overcome cancer" in order to help or to facilitate clinical application and to become the clinical reference.

In the past 60 years, the series of the scientific research achievements and the series of scientific and technological innovations which takes "conquer cancer" as the direction done by us are in this series of "Monographs"; the following thesis or lemma are first proposed internationally, all of which are original papers, internationally pioneered, and have reached the forefront of the world.

XZ-C 's scientific thinking, scientific research design, academic thinking, and scientific dedication about conquering cancer and launching the total cancer attack are summarized as the following monographs:

1. "Walk out of a new road to conquer cancer" (1)(一)

   "Conquer cancer and launch the total attack to cancer – the prevention of cancer and cancer control and cancer treatment at the same level"

2. "Walk out of a new road to conquer cancer" (2) （二）

   "Walking out of a new way of cancer treatment with immune control and regulation of the combination of Chinese and Western medicine"

   (Part I), (Part 2)

3. "Walk out of a new road to conquer cancer" - (3) （三）

   "The research of XZ-C immunomodulation anticancer Chinese medicine"

   ——Experimental research and clinical verification

4. "Walked out of a new road to conquer cancer" – (4)(四)

   "Creating a Science City of Scientific Research Bases with Cancer Multidisciplinary and Cancer related research

   For conquering cancer"

5. "Walked out of a new road to conquer cancer" - (5)(五)

   "The Clinical Application Theory Innovation of 21ˢᵗ Century Cancer Prevention and Treatment Research"

6. "Walked out of a new road to conquer cancer" - (6)(六)

   XZ-C proposes <<to create the Cancer Prevention Research Institute of Environmental Protection >> and to carry out the system engineering of the cancer prevention

   ——Prevention of Pollution and Treatment and Control of Pollution and Prevention of cancer and Anti-cancer anti-cancer

——Dawning prevention cancer research plan and Dawning scientific research spirit

——Medical is benevolence, To set up the moral is the first

7. "Walk out of a new road to conquer cancer" - (7)(七)

"Condense wisdom and conquer cancer - for the benefit of mankind" (part 1), (part 2)

8. "Walk out of a new road to conquer cancer" - (8)(八)

"The Road to overcome cancer"

The library of Prevention of Cancer and Anti-cancer medical research

The Collected Works of Professor Xu Ze (XZ-C)'s Research on Cancer Prevention and Cancer Treatment

XZ-C proposed: How to overcome cancer? How to prevent cancer? How to treat cancer?

XZ-C new concept of cancer treatment

Volume I

<<Conquer Cancer and Launch the total attack to cancer >>
——prevention cancer and cancer control and cancer treatment at the same level and at the same attention and at the same time
The book table or contents or directory (omitted)

Volume II

<<Walked out of a new way of cancer treatment with the immune regulation and control of the combination of Chinese and Western medicine>>
The book table or contents or directory (omitted)

Volume III

<<The research of XZ-C immunomodulation anticancer Chinese medicine ——Experimental research and clinical verification>>
The book table or contents or directory (omitted)

Volume IV

<<To build the science base of multidisciplinary and cancer related research to overcome cancer-Science City>>
Contents (omitted)

Volume V

<<Theoretical Innovation of Cancer Prevention and Management or treatment cancer in the 21st Century>>
Contents (Omitted)

Volume VI

<<XZ-C proposes to create the preventing cancer research institute and to carry out a series of cancer prevention projects>>
Contents (Omitted)
Dawning C plan
Dawning A·B·D plan
Prevention of Cancer and Treatment of Cancer and Preventin of Cancer and anti-cancer
The Dawning Science Research Program
The Dawning Scientific research spirit
Doctor is benevolence, to set up the moral is first

Volume VII

<<Condense Wisdom and Conquer Cancer - Benefiting Mankind>>
Contents (Omitted)
(Volume I and II, which book has two parts)

Volume VIII

<<The Road to Overcome Cancer>>
Directory (omitted)
Volume IX <<On Innovation of Treatment of Cancer>>
Contents (omitted)

Volume X

<<New understanding and new models of cancer treatment>>
Contents (omitted)

Volume XI

"New Concepts and New Methods for Cancer Metastasis Treatment"
Table of Contents (omitted)

Volume XII

"New Progress in Cancer Therapy"
Table of Contents (omitted)

Volume XIII

"New Concepts and New Methods for Cancer Treatment"
Table of Contents (omitted)
[Note: Each volume is a published monograph on cancer medical research]

Note: 1. XZ-C is Xu Ze-China, because science is borderless, but scientists have national and intellectual property.

*2. Cancer is a disaster for all mankind. It must evoke the struggle of the people all over the world. Therefore, there are 8 monographs in the series, which are all in English, distributed worldwide, and published on **Amazon.com, on barnesandnoble.com and on authorhouse.com.***

II. The brief introduction of the experimental and therapy basis of our immune therapy

A. Foreword(1)
B. Foreword(2)
C. Guidance
D. The brief content of Theoretical basis and experimental basis of XZ-C immunomodulation and cancer treatment

A. Foreward (1)

How to overcome cancer, how to prevent cancer by I see
How can I treat cancer *by I see*

XZ-C found problems and raised problems from follow-up results (Hint: how to prevent postoperative recurrence and metastasis is the key to improve long-term outcomes after surgery)

Pathfinding (to overcome cancer, where is the road? How do you find it?)

Pathfinding and footprint (the series of the scientific research results and scientific and technological innovation of cancer prevention and anti-cancer metastasis research)

Published cancer monographs (3 Chinese editions are exclusively distributed nationwide, 5 full English editions are published worldwide)

Participated in the International Congress of Oncology (AACR Academic Conference in USA)

Visiting the Stirling Cancer Institute in Houston, USA (2009)

Accumulated Basic and clinical research on prevention of cancer and anti-cancer metastasis in the past more than 60 years

Accumulated the clinical application experience from more than 12,000 cases in the past more than 34 years

Walked Out of a new road to treat cancer with an immune regulatory and control of the combination of Chinese and Western medicine at the molecular level

Walking out of a new road of cancer treatment to conquer cancer, "Chinese-style anti-cancer", Chinese and Western medicine combined with immune regulation and control

- Published the English monograph «The Road to Overcome Cancer»

- December 6, 2016, published in Washington, DC, global distribution, Amazon website and Barnesandnoble.com and Authorhouse.com
- Published the English monograph "Condense Wisdom and Conquer Cancer"

-Published in December 2017 (volume 1), published in February 2018 (the next volume), published in Washington, USA, full English version, global distribution, Amazon website and Barnesandnoble.com and Authorhouse.com.
- Published the English monograph "Conquer Cancer and launch The Total Attack to Cancer" – cancer prevention and cancer control and cancer treatment at the same level and at the same attention)

In November 2018, the United States published in Washington, DC, and the Amazon website and Barnesandnoble.com and Authorhouse.com

"Walked out of the new way of cancer treatment with immune control and regulation of the combination of Chinese and Western medicine"

- How to overcome cancer? How to treat cancer?
  Walked out of the new road to conquer cancer
  XZ-C new concept of cancer treatment
  (Volume 1), (2)

1. How did we find the new way of treatment of cancer with the immune regulation and control?

In the past 30 years, we have achieved a series of scientific research achievements, scientific and technological innovation from our science research work which took "conquer cancer" as the research direction and the road which we looked for a road to conquer cancer is in this way to come over a step by step:

(1) New findings from the follow-up results: we should look for ways to prevent recurrence and metastasis after prevention and treatment.
(2) New findings from experimental results of cancer animal models: looking for ways to prevent thymic atrophy, promote thymic hyperplasia, enhance the path of immunity, find the way of immune reconstruction, and propose a new concept of immune regulation and treatment of cancer.
(3) The key to studying cancer treatment is anti-metastasis: looking for ways to eliminate cancer cells on the way to metastasis, and put forward the new concept of the cancer treatment "two points and one line theory", not only paying attention to two points, but also cutting off one line.

2. Why should we take a new path of treatment of cancer with immune regulation and control?

This answer or it is because of the new finding from our laboratory experimental research:

(1) Resection of the thymus can produce a cancer-bearing animal model
(2) Experimental results suggest that metastasis is related to immune function and when the immune function is low, cancer metastasis can be promoted.
(3) The experimental results showed that the host thymus was acutely progressively atrophied after inoculation of cancer cells, cell proliferation was blocked, and the volume was significantly reduced.
(4) The experimental results showed that when the experimental mice were inoculated with cancer cells, the solid tumors were cut to the length of the thumb. After one week, the thymus was found to have no progressive atrophy.

The results of our laboratory experiments showed that the thymus of the cancer-bearing mice showed progressive atrophy, reduced volume, blocked cell proliferation, decreased mature cells, and low immune function. By the end of the tumor, the thymus is extremely atrophied and the texture becomes hard. Therefore, it is necessary to prevent thymus atrophy, to perform the immune regulation and control, and immune reconstitution. Therefore, we must take a new path of treatment of cancer with the immune regulation and control.

3. What is the theoretical basis and experimental basis for taking the new path of treatment of cancer with the immune regulation and control?

From the above experimental studies it was found that: thymus atrophy and low immune function may be one of the cancer pathogenesis and pathogenesis, so its treatment principle must be to prevent thymic atrophy and to promote thymocyte proliferation and to increase immune function.

The immune function of the body, especially cellular immune function, T lymphocyte function, and the immune regulation function of the thymus should be explored at the molecular level to search the methods for immune regulation and control and the effective drug research should be sought.

About the effect of tumor on the thymus: The experimental results show that after inoculation of cancer cells, the thymus is immediately suppressed, and the whole process is progressively atrophy, so the thymus quickly loses the tumor immune effect. It was observed in the experiment that the thymus gland changed its morphological structure shortly after inoculation of the cancer cells, and the whole course of disease showed progressive atrophy. **By the end of the tumor, the weight of the thymus was reduced from 78.13±13.2 mg to 20±5 mg, and the volume was reduced from 5 to 8 mm in diameter to 1 mm, and cell proliferation was significantly blocked.**

Due to progressive atrophy of the thymus, cell proliferation is blocked, mature cells are reduced or depleted, cell viability is decreased, and thymus hormone secretion is also reduced. The cellular immune function of the body is inevitably damaged. The mouse's defense ability is low and the transplanted cancer cells have a large number of growth and reproduction or grow greatly and multiply.

The thymus is an important central lymphoid organ that promotes T cell differentiation and maturation to exert cellular immunity and complement B cells to produce antibodies. The thymus also produces a variety of thymus hormones that promote the differentiation and maturation of immune lymphocyte stem cells.

In the late stage, due to the progression of the tumor, a large number of immunosuppressive factors are produced, thereby losing the positive effect of anti-tumor immunity.

As a result of the above experimental studies, it was found that the thymus of the cancer-bearing mice showed progressive atrophy, and the function of the central immune organ was impaired, the immune function was decreased, and the immune surveillance was low. Therefore, the treatment principle must be to prevent the thymus from shrinking and

promote thymic hyperplasia and protect bone hematopoiesis, enhance immune surveillance, and control immune escape from malignant cells. Therefore, XZ-C proposed that immune regulation should be used to treat cancer.

4. How should I perform immunomodulatory therapy?

There are two ways:

1) By immunorecombination through human immune cell transplantation, transplantation of embryonic thymocytes in mice can be carried out in the laboratory, but it is not feasible in the human body, because the thymus is a human growth and development organ, which is irreplaceable and thus cannot be implemented.

2) Chinese medication has a large number of prescriptions to regulate immune function, especially the beneficial or tonic Chinese medicine generally has the effect of regulating immune activity or in particular, Chinese medicines for tonics generally have the effect of regulating immune activity, showing the correlation between dose and effect or benefit under general experimental condition. Under the general experimental conditions, the correlation between dose and benefit is presented, and the Chinese medicine of tonic is more significant in improving the immunity of the body.

5. Why is Chinese medication used? Why is it looked for from Chinese medication?

It is because western medicine which can boost immune drugs is rarely and Chinese medicine has a large number of prescriptions to boost immunity. In particular, polysaccharides and tonics have the effect of regulating immune activity.

In the past 34 years, our laboratory has carried out a series of experimental studies to find new anti-cancer and anti-metastatic drugs from natural medicines and look for the anti-cancer drugs to prevent thymic atrophy and to increase immune function and look for the new anti-cancer drugs from the nature medicine; to look for anti-metastatic, anti-recurrence drugs; look for drugs that inhibit only cancer cells but not normal cells; look for the drugs which have prevention of thymic atrophy and adjust the regulatory relationship between the host and the tumor and prevent recurrence and metastasis from traditional Chinese medicine.

6. How did our laboratory conduct experimental research on screening anticancer and anti-metastatic drugs from traditional Chinese medicine?

(1) Using the method of in vitro culture of cancer cells to conduct screening experiments on the rate of cancer suppression of Chinese herbal medicines:

In vitro screening test: The cancer cells were cultured in vitro to observe the direct damage of the drug to cancer cells.

In-tube screening test: In the test tube for culturing cancer cells, the raw crude drug (500 ug/ml) was separately placed to observe whether it inhibited the cancer cells. We used 200 kinds of Chinese herbal medicines that traditional Chinese medicine believed to have anti-cancer effects. Screening experiments were performed in vitro. The toxicity of the drug to the cells was tested by normal fiber cell culture under the same conditions and then compared.

(2) Making animal models of cancer-bearing animals, and conducting experimental screening of Chinese herbal medicines on the rate of cancer suppression in cancer-bearing animals

In vivo anti-cancer screening test, 240 mice per batch were divided into 8 groups, 30 in each group, the 7th group was the blank control group, the 8th group was treated with 5-F or CTX as the control group, and the whole group was vaccinated with EAC or S180 or H22 cancer cells. After inoculation for 24 hours, each rat was orally fed with crude biological powder and long-term feeding of the traditional Chinese medicine was used to observe the survival period, toxicity and side effects and the survival rate was calculated, and the cancer inhibition rate was calculated.

In this way, we conducted a four-year experimental study.

The experimental study on the pathogenesis, metastasis and recurrence mechanism and an experimental study of how tumors cause host death of tumor-bearing mice for 3 years was carried out. More than 1,000 tumor-bearing animal models are used each year. A total of nearly 6,000 tumor-bearing animal models were made in 4 years. Pathological anatomy of the liver, spleen, lung, thymus, and kidney was performed after the death of each experimental mouse. A total of more than 20,000 slices were made. To find out if there are tiny pathogens that may be carcinogenic. Tumor microvessel establishment and microcirculation of 100 tumor-bearing mice were observed by microcirculation microscopy.

Through experimental research, we have found for the first time in China that the traditional Chinese medicine TG has obvious effects in inhibiting tumor microvessel formation. It has been used in more than 80 patients in clinical anti-metastatic treatment.

Experimental results:

Among the 200 kinds of Chinese herbal medicines screened by animal experiments in our laboratory, 48 species were selected, and even excellent, inhibited the proliferation of cancer cells, and the tumor inhibition rate was above 75-90%. However, there are also some commonly used traditional Chinese medicines that are generally considered to have anti-cancer effects. After screening for animal tumors in vitro and in vivo, there is no anti-cancer effect, or the effect is very small. In this group, 152 kinds of anti-cancer effects were eliminated by animal experiments.

The 48 kinds of traditional Chinese medicines with good cancer suppression rate were selected by this experiment, and then the optimized combination was repeated to carry out the cancer suppression experiment in vivo. Finally, the XZ-C1-10 (Xu Ze-China) immune regulation anti-cancer series was formed. Traditional Chinese medicine, from experimental

research to clinical verification, is applied to clinical practice on the basis of the success of animal experiments. After 20 years of clinical trials of more than 12,000 clinical cases, the curative effect is remarkable, which is independent innovation, independent invention and independent intellectual property rights.

The purpose is to screen out new drugs for anti-cancer, anti-metastatic, and immune-enhanced immune regulation and control with no drug resistance, no toxic side effects, and high selectivity and which can be used for long-term orally.

Because:

(1) **We should give full play of China's advantages in areas where China has advantages. In the field of cancer research, traditional Chinese medicine is an advantage of China. We should play this advantage in cancer research and explore and develop effective Chinese herbal medicines for cancer prevention and anti-cancer.**

In-depth research should be carried out to analyze and purify the active ingredients; to carry out research on the immunological pharmacology of traditional Chinese medicine; to carry out research on molecular level and gene level, so that the modernization of Chinese herbal medicines is in line with international standards.

(2) The combination of Chinese and Western medicine is the characteristic and advantage of Chinese medicine. It comes from Chinese medicine, higher than Chinese medicine. It comes from Western medicine, higher than Western medicine, and is a combination of Chinese medicine and Western medicine. 1+ 1=2,2>1, which makes the treatment of cancer combined with Chinese and Western medicine more perfect and reasonable, and improves the curative effect. Because traditional cancer therapy (surgery, radiotherapy, chemotherapy) reduces the body's immune function, and immune regulation and anti-cancer drugs increase the body's immune function, and become a comprehensive treatment, post-operative immunization, radiotherapy, Chinese medicine immunization (immunotherapy), chemotherapy Chinese medicine immunization (immunotherapy chemotherapy), its efficacy will inevitably increase.

1) Why is Chinese herbal medicine the advantage of China in cancer research?
It is because treatment must be directed to the cause, pathogenesis, pathophysiology.

The following multidisciplinary and canceric relationships should be sought for treatments, drugs:

a. cancer and immunity have a positive relationship, should look for immunomodulatory drugs;
b. some cancers have a positive relationship with the virus, should look for antiviral drugs;
c. some cancers have a positive relationship with endocrine hormones, should look for drugs that regulate endocrine hormones;

15

  d. some cancers are related to fungi, and anti-fungal drugs should be sought;
  e. Some cancers are associated with chronic inflammation and should be searched for drugs that are resistant to chronic inflammation.

These immune regulation, adjustment of endocrine hormones, anti-virus, etc., are rare in modern medicine and western medicine. However, China's Fuzheng Guben and Buxu Chinese herbal medicines are rich in resources, and have immune regulation, hormone adjustment, and anti-virus. Good function, and has a long history and clinical application experience and works. In recent years, some researchers and graduate students have carried out some experimental analysis and research on the molecular level of Chinese herbal medicine. It should be said that in the study of cancer, the richness of Chinese herbal medicine resources is an advantage.

2) Why is Chinese herbal medicine the advantage of China in the field of cancer research?

Our experiments have the following experimental evidence and their own clinically validated data accumulation.

It is because our laboratory has screened out 48 Chinese herbal medicines that have a good anti-tumor rate.

Existing anticancer drugs not only kill cancer cells but also normal cells, and have large adverse reactions. We have tried new cancer drugs in cancer-bearing mice to find new drugs that inhibit cancer cells without affecting normal cells. We spent a full three years on the anti-tumor screening experiments of cancer-bearing animals in 200 kinds of Chinese herbal medicines used in traditional anti-cancer prescriptions and anti-cancer agents reported in various places. As a result, 48 strains were screened for better tumor inhibition.

3) Why is Chinese herbal medicine the advantage of China in cancer research?

It is because our laboratory finds from the Chinese herbal medicine to promote thymic hyperplasia, prevent thymus atrophy, and improve the immune regulation of traditional Chinese medicine.

We conducted a full 4 years of oncology research work in the laboratory. Our laboratory experimental results showed that the thymus of the cancer-bearing mice showed progressive atrophy, the volume was reduced, the cell proliferation was blocked, and the mature cells were reduced. By the end of the tumor, the thymus is extremely atrophied and the texture becomes hard.

From the above experimental studies, it is found that thymus atrophy and low immune function may be one of the pathogenic factors and pathogenesis of tumors, so it is necessary to try to prevent thymus atrophy, promote thymocyte proliferation, and increase immunity. The immune function of the body, especially cellular immunity, the function of T lymphocytes, and the immune regulation function of the thymus should be explored at the molecular level, and methods for immune regulation and effective drug research should be sought.

How should we find new ways to regulate immune therapy?

The anti-cancer immunity of traditional Chinese medicine polysaccharides is progressing rapidly. A large number of immunopharmacological studies have been carried out at the molecular level. Polysaccharides can improve the body's immune surveillance system, including natural killer cells (NK), macrophages (MΦ), and killer T cells (CTL).), T cells, LAK cells, tumor infiltrating lymphocytes (TIL), interleukin (IL) and other cytokines are active to kill tumor cells.

Traditional Chinese medicine and western medicine have their own strengths, each with its own shortness. Compared with Western medicine immunopharmacology, traditional Chinese medicine immunopharmacology has its own characteristics and advantages, and each has its own shortcomings. The advantage of traditional Chinese medicine immunology is that a large number of Chinese medicines have the effect of regulating the body's immune function. The Chinese medicine is rich in source and is an effective medicine for long-term clinical treatment. After extraction, it may obtain active ingredients and obvious pharmacological effects (including immunomodulatory effects). The research process saves people time and has high efficiency.

As mentioned above, in the field of cancer treatment, Chinese herbal medicine is China's advantage. In the past 28 years, the experimental research of our Experimental Surgery Research Institute and the clinical specialization of oncology clinics have confirmed the clinical trials in a large number of cases. It is confirmed that in the treatment of cancer, Chinese herbal medicine is China. The advantages can go international and benefit patients. Many cancer patients have significantly prolonged their survival.

7. Why should we take the road of combining Chinese and Western medicine to treat cancer?

(1) It is because the combination of Chinese and Western medicine is the characteristics and advantages of Chinese medicine. Both Chinese and Western medicines have their own strengths, and each has its own shortcomings. The two should complement each other's strengths, combine innovation, innovate "Chinese medicine", and innovate "Chinese-style anti-cancer."

Innovation is not only technology and product innovation, but also basic theoretical innovation. Theoretical innovation is the greatest achievement. Scientific development is based on the innovation of basic theory, which is the biggest innovation.

The combination of Chinese and Western medicine is the characteristics and advantages of Chinese medicine. The goal of combining Chinese and Western medicine should be combined with innovation. The goal of combining innovation should be to improve the clinical medical effect. The standard of efficacy of cancer patients is: cancer patients have long survival time, good quality of life, and no complications.

Because of the combination of Chinese and Western medicine, it comes from Chinese medicine, higher than Chinese medicine; from Western medicine, higher than Western medicine, 1+1=2, 2>1. This is for the Chinese to use, the ancient for the present, to modernize Chinese medicine, to the forefront of the international. It is because Chinese medicine is the essence of Chinese culture.

> (2) How to combine Chinese and Western medicine? The advantages of traditional Chinese medicine and western medicine should be combined to improve the level and efficacy of cancer treatment.

1) From the results of follow-up, it was found that postoperative recurrence and metastasis were the key factors affecting the long-term efficacy of surgery. Therefore, we also ask us an important question: clinicians must pay attention to and study the prevention and treatment measures for postoperative recurrence and metastasis in order to improve long-term efficacy after surgery.

I reviewed my 60 years of clinical medical practice cases and followed up, then analyzed, reflected on successful experiences, failed lessons, and realized a truth: conquering cancer requires updating concepts, updating thinking, and updating concepts, having Innovation, in the urgent issue of cancer research, looking for clinical breakthroughs in the weak links of modern medical medicine, recognizing that the technology of surgical resection of tumors in the 20th century has achieved brilliant achievements. The next research goal and task of surgeons is not only to further study excellence. Good radical surgery, and should prevent postoperative recurrence and metastasis. To further improve the long-term efficacy of radical surgery.

At present, the removal of tumors together with regional lymphatic vessels and lymph nodes does not prevent the transfer of blood, as well as the dissemination and shedding of blood, cell planting and dissemination. **Therefore, the research work of tumor surgeons, the next research goal should be the experimental and clinical research on radical recurrence, metastasis prevention and treatment**, that is, the early 21st century should be a century of brilliant achievements in prevention and treatment of postoperative recurrence and metastasis. **If the problem of postoperative recurrence and metastasis is not solved, the long-term effect of surgery on cancer treatment will not achieve satisfactory results.**

Therefore, the surgical goal of the 21st century should be the prevention and treatment of recurrence and metastasis after radical cancer.

2) to prevent postoperative recurrence and metastasis of cancer should start from the surgery.

The surgical technique of cancer surgery is extremely important. It is necessary to prevent the operation of the cancer cells from causing or causing the blood vessels to metastasize, preventing the spread of intraoperative cancer cells and preventing cancer cells from growing.

Do a good tumor-free technique for radical cancer surgery to prevent intraoperative dissemination, metastasis, implantation, and missed diagnosis.

Tumor-free techniques are extremely important and should prevent surgical procedures from causing or causing cancer cells to metastasize.

At the time of surgery, it must be noted that all techniques are conducive to preventing the metastasis of cancer cells, and do not promote or increase the chance of cancer cell metastasis, resulting in iatrogenic transfer and dissemination. Surgical removal of tumors, regardless of the size of the surgery, must pay attention to and adhere to the concept of no tumor and tumor-free technology. Surgeons must establish the concept of both no tumor and sterility, the concept of both tumor-free technology and aseptic technique, even the tumor-free technology is stricter than the aseptic technique. **In the operation, one knife and one cut, one needle and one thread, and even each operation has the possibility of promoting cancer metastasis. This possibility is caused by the operator's excessive compression, needle wear, knife cutting and other adverse operations on the tumor tissue. Increasingly, these possibilities for the implantation, spread and metastasis of iatrogenic cancer cells by the surgical procedure itself have been confirmed by molecular biology or immunohistochemistry. In some patients, cancer cells can be found in the circulation around** the bloodstream during surgery, or from the negative of the cancer cells before the operation to the positive after the operation, indicating that the operation may cause the spread of cancer cells. Therefore, all tumor surgery, cutting must pay attention to tumor-free technology.

Prevention and treatment of postoperative recurrence and metastasis:

1) **To carry out research on the combination of Chinese and Western medicine, immunotherapy** and cancer treatment, traditional Chinese medicine immunopharmacology research, immunotherapy, immune prevention, prolong survival, and improve long-term efficacy.
2) Intraoperative application of immunoregulatory Chinese medicine, because cancer patients are immune function is low, are applied with immune Chinese medicine, in order to facilitate postoperative recovery, and prevent postoperative recurrence and metastasis.

In summary, therefore, we should take a new path of combining Chinese and Western medicine with immune regulation and treatment. We have found a way to control cancer, take a new road combining Chinese and Western medicine, and take a new path of combining Chinese and Western medicine with cancer at the molecular level.

B. Foreword (2)

In 1985, I conducted a petition with more than 3,000 patients who underwent radical surgery for various cancers. It was found that most patients had recurrence and metastasis 2 to 3 years after surgery, and some even metastasized several months after surgery. This made me realize that although the operation is successful, the long-term efficacy is not satisfactory. Postoperative recurrence and metastasis are the key factors affecting the long-term efficacy of the operation. It also reminds us that prevention and treatment of postoperative recurrence and metastasis is the key to prolonging postoperative survival. Therefore, basic research must be carried out, and without breakthroughs in basic research, clinical efficacy is difficult to improve. So we established the Institute of Experimental Surgery and spent a total of 24 years conducting a series of experimental research and clinical validation work from the following three aspects.

First, explore the mechanism of cancer onset, invasion and recurrence and metastasis, and carry out experimental research on effective measures to regulate invasion, recurrence and metastasis.

We have been conducting laboratory research for a full four years in the laboratory. They are clinical basic research and research projects. They are all clinically raised questions to explain these clinical problems or solve these clinical problems through experimental research.

Second, look for new anti-cancer, anti-metastatic, anti-recurrence new drug experimental research from natural drugs.

The existing anticancer drugs kill both cancer cells and normal cells, and have large adverse reactions. We used anti-tumor experiments in cancer-bearing mice to find new drugs that only inhibit cancer cells without affecting normal cells. We spent a full three years on the anti-tumor screening experiments of cancer-bearing animals in 200 kinds of Chinese herbal medicines used in traditional anti-cancer prescriptions and anti-cancer agents reported in various places. RESULTS: 48 kinds of traditional Chinese medicines with good anti-tumor effect and good ascending effect were screened out, and the traditional Chinese medicine Huang Lateng ethyl acetate extract (TG) which can inhibit the new microvessels was found out.

Third, clinical verification work

Through the above four years to explore the basic experimental research of recurrence and metastasis mechanism, and after three years of experimental research from natural drugs, we have identified a batch of XZ-C1-10 immunomodulatory anticancer Chinese medicine, and passed more than 12,000 cases in 20 years. The clinical verification of patients with advanced metastasis or postoperative metastasis, XZ-C immunomodulation of anticancer traditional Chinese medicine, has achieved good results, can improve the quality of life of patients, improve patient symptoms, and significantly prolong the survival of patients.

Through the review, analysis, reflection and experience of my clinical practice cases for more than 60 years, combined with the results and findings of my experimental research on tumor-bearing animals for more than 34 years, in January 2001, Hubei Science and Technology Press published a new understanding of cancer treatment. And the new model, published in January 2006 by the People's Medical Publishing House, "New Concepts and New Methods for Cancer Metastasis Treatment", which was also awarded "Three by the General Administration of Press and Publication of the People's Republic of China in April 2007" with one hundred "Original Book Award.

This book is a true record of the author's scientific thinking from "experiment to clinical, then clinical to experimental." The summary of experimental research and clinical verification data has risen to the theoretical essence, and proposes new discoveries and new understandings, such as clinical practical oncology theory, cancer treatment, research development and reform, and these clinical practical innovation theories can be used to guide Clinical treatment work.

The theoretical innovation of clinical application is because all clinical treatment, medication, and diagnosis must have a reasonable theoretical basis. More than 50 years of clinical tumor surgery practice has made me deeply understand that because the etiology, pathogenesis and pathophysiology of tumors are not well understood, "oncology" has become one of the most backward developments in medical science, and more basic scientific research, clinical validation research, and a combination of basic and clinical research needs further to be done.

In the past 7 years, a series of clinical basic experimental research and basic problems have been explored on more than 6,000 tumor-bearing animal models, and 200 kinds of Chinese herbal medicines have been screened for tumor-inhibiting tumor-inhibiting experiments in vivo. These were completed by several graduate students. . "Exploring the effect of spleen on tumor growth and the anti-cancer effect of Jianpi Yiqi Decoction" was completed by Master Zhu Siping: "Experimental study on the combined transplantation of fetal liver, spleen and thymocytes for the treatment of malignant tumors" by Zou Shaomin The Ph.D. completed: "Experimental study on the anti-tumor effect of Fuzheng Peiben on S180 mice" was completed by Master Li Zhengxun: "Experimental study on the inhibitory effect of ethyl acetate extract (TG) on the neovascularization of transplanted tumors in mice", by Liu Yu master completed. The topics of the master's and doctoral students are the sub-topics of my total research project, and they are the basic issues closely related to clinical practice. The graduate students have carried out and completed a lot of hard and meticulous experimental research work, contributing to the development of anti-cancer, anti-cancer and experimental oncology medicine.

The content of this book includes experimental research and clinically validated cases, as well as new concepts, new theories and new models of cancer treatment that have been promoted to theory. Some of the insights are first proposed for originality. In the spirit of "Hundred Flowers Blossom", we update our thinking and change our concept to enlighten us. Ideas and further innovation. Due to the rapid development of oncology medicine, and involving many disciplines such as molecular biology, molecular immunology, genetic engineering, etc., there are a wide range of knowledge. If there are errors or omissions in the book, please ask colleagues, experts and readers for your advice.

C. Guidance

Enlightenment or Inspiration from "Walked out of A New Way of Cancer Treatment with Immune regulation and control of the Combination of Chinese Medicine and Western Medicine"

———Proposed the theoretical basis and experimental basis of treatment of Cancer with immune regulation and control

Inspiration of the research from walked out of a new road: **pathfinding**

Where is the road of conquering cancer? How to find this way?

How did the road come over? The cause is that the path-finding is a step-by-step and hard trek, hard to climb, after 60 years of hard work which took "conquer cancer" as the research direction to overcome cancer research, step by step a scientific research footprint came over.

Mr. Lu Xun said: "There is no way in the world. If there are more people going, they will go out of the way."

Why should we take a new path of cancer treatment with immune regulation and control? Why should we take the new path of cancer treatment with combination of Chinese and Western medicine? Why should we take the new path of cancer treatment with combination of Chinese and Western medicine at the molecular level? What is the theoretical basis and experimental basis for taking immunoregulation cancer treatment? Why do you look for an experimental study of new drugs against cancer and metastasis and recurrence from natural medicines?

Pathfinding – looking for ways to overcome cancer, where is the road?

What we have found is a path of immune regulation and control treatment of cancer, taking a new road combining Chinese and Western medicine, and taking a new path of combining traditional Chinese medicine and western medicine at the molecular level.

The road is such a step by step, difficult to trek, after 60 years of hard work to overcome cancer research, step by step a scientific research footprint:

- navigate
- Path finding and research footprint
- *Walked out of a new path of XZ-C immune regulation and control at the molecular level, Western medicine combined with new cancer treatment*
- The theoretical system *of cancer treatment with XZ-C immunoregulation has been formed, which is the theoretical basis and experimental basis for cancer immunotherapy*
- The series products and adaptation range of XZ-C immune regulation and *control anti-cancer Chinese medicine*
- *XZ-C immunomodulation anticancer Chinese medicine is the result of the modernization of traditional Chinese medicine*

D. Theoretical basis and experimental basis of cancer treatment of XZ-C immunomodulation regulation and control

1. New findings of follow-up results

This is a new discovery from the clinical follow-up results, from the clinical to provide issues and to find problems, but the following series of experimental basic research and clinical validation observations were performed:

Cause:

(1)   Why do I study cancer? I am a clinical surgeon, why do you study cancer? This was due to the results of a group of patients who had a postoperative visit to a cancer patient.

In 1985, I conducted a petition with more than 3,000 patients who underwent radical surgery for various cancers outside the chest (all according to the operating room registration list).

It was found that most patients relapsed and metastasized 2 to 3 years after surgery. This made me realize that although the operation is successful, the long-term efficacy is not satisfactory. Postoperative recurrence and metastasis are the key factors affecting the long-term efficacy of the operation. It also reminds us that prevention and treatment of postoperative recurrence and metastasis is the key to prolonging postoperative survival.

Therefore, clinical basic research must be carried out. Without breakthroughs in basic research, clinical efficacy is difficult to improve, so we established the Institute of Experimental Surgery and conducted a series of experimental research and clinical validation work.

(2)   From the results of follow-up, it was found that:

1.   postoperative recurrence and metastasis are the key factors affecting the long-term efficacy of surgery;
2.   prompt clinicians must pay attention to and study the prevention and treatment of postoperative recurrence and metastasis, in order to improve the long-term effect of surgery, so we established an experimental surgical laboratory, conducted experimental tumor research, performed cancer cell transplantation, established a tumor animal model, and carried out A series of experimental tumor studies: Explored the mechanism and regularity of cancer recurrence and metastasis;

Explored the relationship between tumors and immune and immune organs, as well as immune organs and tumors;

Explored methods for suppressing progressive atrophy of immune organs and rebuilding immunity when tumor progression is inhibited; searched for effective measures to regulate cancer invasion, recurrence, and metastasis; the anti-cancer Chinese herbal medicines commonly used in 200 literatures were tested for the anti-tumor rate of cancer-bearing solid tumors; Looking for new experimental studies of anticancer, anti-metastasis and anti-recurrence from natural medicines; using modern science and technology, in-depth study of the discovery of prevention of cancer and anti-cancer Chinese herbal medicine. In the anti-cancer Chinese herbal medicine, the traditional anti-cancer Chinese herbal medicine was tested in a strict, scientific and repeated tumor-bearing animal model and eliminated the effect without stability, 48 kinds of Z-C immunoregulatory anticancer Chinese medicines with good curative effect were screened out. It has been applied to clinical practice on the basis of the success of animal experiments. After 30 years of clinical trials of a large number of clinical cases, the curative effect is remarkable.

2. New findings in animal experiment research

From the experimental tumor research findings, in order to explore the cause, pathogenesis, invasion and metastasis mechanism of cancer, and find effective measures for regulation, intervention, invasion, recurrence and metastasis, the author and colleagues conducted a full four-year experimental tumor research work.

(1) Experiment 1: Excision of mouse thymus (Thymus, TH) to produce a tumor-bearing animal model, injection of immunosuppressive drugs contributes to the establishment of a cancer-bearing animal model. The research conclusions show that the occurrence and development of cancer have a significant correlation with the thymus and function of the host immune organs.

(2) Experiment 2: Whether it is low immune first and then easy to get cancer, or cancer occurs first and then low immunity, the experimental results confirmed that the first immune system is low and then easy to have cancer occurrence and development, if no immune function is low, it is not easy to vaccinate success. The experimental results suggest that improving and maintaining good immune function, and protecting the central immune organ thymus is one of the important measures to prevent cancer.

(3) Experiment 3: In the study of the relationship between cancer metastasis and immunity, an animal model of liver metastasis was established and divided into two groups, A and B groups. Group A used immunosuppressive drugs, and group B did not. Results The number of intrahepatic metastases in group A was significantly higher than that in group B. The experimental results suggest that metastasis is associated with immunity, low immune function or the use of immunosuppressive drugs can promote tumor metastasis.

(4) Experiment 4: When investigating the effect of tumor on immune organs, it was found that with the progress of cancer, the thymus showed progressive atrophy, and the host thymus was acute progressive atrophy after inoculation of cancer cells, and cell proliferation was blocked. The volume is significantly reduced. The experimental results suggest that the tumor may inhibit the thymus and cause the immune organs to shrink.

(5) Experiment 5: It was found in the experiment that some of the experimental mice did not have a successful vaccination or the tumor grew very small, and the thymus did not significantly shrink. To understand the relationship between tumor and thymus atrophy, a group of experimental mice transplanted solid tumors were resected when they reached the size of the thumb. After 1 month of dissection, it was found that the thymus did not undergo atrophy. Therefore, we speculate that a solid tumor may produce a factor that is not yet known to inhibit the thymus, which needs further study.

From experimental tumor research it was found:

(1) Resection of the thymus (Thymus, TH) can produce a cancer-bearing animal model;
(2) The experimental results suggest that metastasis is related to immunity, and low immune function may promote tumor metastasis;

(3)   The experimental results showed that the host thymus was acutely progressively atrophied after inoculation of the tumor cells, the cell proliferation was blocked, and the volume was significantly reduced;

(4)   The experimental results showed that when the transplanted solid tumor of the experimental mouse grew to a large thumb, it was removed. After one week, the thymus was found to have no atrophy.

From the above experimental studies, it is found that thymus atrophy and immune dysfunction may be one of the pathogenesis factors and pathogenesis of tumors. We should take the immune function from the body, especially cellular immunity, T lymphocyte function and thymus immune regulation function in the molecule. Explore the level and seek ways to regulate immune.

In order to explore the etiology, pathogenesis and pathophysiology of cancer, we conducted a series of animal experiments, from the results of experimental research to analyze and think, so that we can obtain new discoveries, new thinking, new enlightenment: one of the causes of cancer It may be atrophy of the thymus, impaired thymus function, and low immune function. Therefore, Professor Xu Ze mentioned one of the causes and pathogenesis of cancer at international conferences, which may be thymus atrophy, impaired central immune organ function, low immune function, decreased immune surveillance ability and immune escape. But what is the cause of the host's thymus atrophy? After repeated thinking and speculation, it may be because a factor produced by solid tumors inhibits the thymus, but this needs further experimental research, we can temporarily call it "cancer Thymus inhibition or suppressive factor".

Looking back on the research history of cancer in the past 100 years, the research on the etiology, pathophysiology and pathogenesis of cancer is still rare. In the past 100 years, people have made efforts in clinical research and pathological research of cancer in the fields of surgery, radiotherapy and chemotherapy. Laboratory basic research and clinical basic research such as mutation, cloning, proliferation, metastasis, and planting regularity, such as invasion, metastasis, tumor thrombus, immunity, and endocrine, are relatively rare. Many large hospitals have not established laboratories for clinical basic research. Reviewing and reflecting on the experience and lessons of the author's clinical surgery for more than 60 years, it is clear that without clinical breakthroughs, clinical efficacy is difficult to improve.

3. The animal experiment enlightenment: the theoretical basis and experimental basis of "protecting Thymus and increasing immune function of XZ-C immune regulation and control cancer therapy"

The author's laboratory found that the thymus of the cancer-bearing mice showed progressive atrophy, and the central immune organs were damaged, and should be protected by "protecting Thymus and increasing Immune function."

Based on the implications of experimental research on the etiology and pathogenesis of cancer, Professor Xu Ze first proposed a new theory and method for XZ-C immunomodulation targeted therapy. As a result of experimental research, it was found that the thymus of the cancer-bearing mice showed progressive atrophy, and the central immune organ function

was impaired, the immune function was decreased, and the immune surveillance was low. Therefore, the treatment principle must be to prevent progressive atrophy of the thymus and promote thymic hyperplasia and to protect bone marrow hematopoietic function, to improve immune surveillance, and to control immune escape of malignant cells.

It is well known that immune organs have central immune organs and peripheral immune organs. The former includes the thymus and bone marrow, and the latter includes the spleen and lymph nodes. Now It has been confirmed that **when cancer occurs, a factor that suppresses immune organs [we temporarily call it a cancer suppressor Thymus (TH) factor] inhibits the thymus, causes the thymus to gradually shrink, the central immune function is inhibited, and the immune function declines. To make the immune surveillance weakened or missing, the tumor will inevitably develop further.**

After 34 years of clinical trials and observations of more than 12,000 patients with advanced cancer in the oncology clinic, the author has confirmed that the treatment principle of breast enhancement is correct and reasonable, and the curative effect is satisfactory.

XZ-C (XU ZE-China) immunomodulatory therapy was first proposed by Professor Xu Ze in China in 2006 in his book "New Concepts and New Methods for Cancer Metastasis Treatment". He believes that under normal circumstances, there is a dynamic balance between cancer and body defense. The occurrence and development of cancer is caused by the imbalance of dynamic balance. If the state of the disorder has been adjusted to a normal level, the growth of the cancer can be controlled and allowed to subside.

It is well known that the occurrence and development of cancer and its prognosis are determined by the comparison of two factors, namely, the biological characteristics of cancer cells and the host body's own ability to control cancer cells. If the balance between the two is cancer, the cancer can be controlled. Unbalance is the development of cancer.

Under normal circumstances, the host's body itself has certain restrictions on cancer cells, but in the case of cancer, these restrictive defenses will be inhibited and damaged to varying degrees, resulting in cancer cells losing immune surveillance and cancer cell immune function escape, allowing cancer cells to further develop and metastasize.

It should protect, regulate and activate the anti-cancer immune system in human body.

4. Pathfinding: an experimental study of finding new anticancer drugs from natural drugs

The study of searching for and screening new anti-cancer and anti-metastatic drugs from traditional Chinese medicine:

The purpose is to screen out new and anti-cancer drugs of anti-cancer, anti-metastatic, anti-recurrent that have no drug resistance, no toxic side effects, and high selectivity, and which can be taken for a long-term orally.

It is a scientific research design, and plans to find new anticancer drugs from natural drugs through animal experiments in cancer-bearing mice, and to find anti-metastatic and anti-relapsing drugs. To find a traditional Chinese medicine that inhibits only cancer cells without inhibiting normal cells, and seeks new drugs to control metastasis, adjust the regulatory relationship between the host and the tumor, and prevent recurrence.

To this end, our laboratory conducted the following experimental studies to screen new anticancer and anti-metastatic drugs from traditional Chinese medicine:

(1)   Using the method of in vitro culture of cancer cells to conduct screening experiments on the rate of cancer suppression of Chinese herbal medicines:

In vitro screening test: The cancer cells were cultured in vitro to observe the direct damage of the drug to cancer cells.

In-tube screening test, in the test tube of cultured cancer cells, respectively, into the crude drug product (500ug / ml), to observe whether it has a tumor suppressor effect on cancer cells, we will traditional Chinese medicine think that there are 200 kinds of Chinese herbal medicines with anti-cancer effect, An in vitro screening test was performed one by one. The toxicity of the drug to the cells was tested by normal fiber cell culture under the same conditions and then compared.

(2)   Making animal models of cancer-bearing animals, and conducting experimental screening of Chinese herbal medicines on the rate of cancer suppression in cancer-bearing animals

In vivo anti-cancer screening test: 240 mice in each batch were divided into 8 groups, 30 in each group, the 7th group was the blank control group, the 8th group was treated with 5-F or CTX as the control group, and the whole group of mice Inoculate EAC or S180 or H22 cancer cells. After inoculation for 24 hours, each rat was orally fed with crude drug powder, and the traditional Chinese medicine was screened for a long time. The survival time, toxicity and side effects were calculated, the survival rate was calculated, and the cancer inhibition rate was calculated.

In this way, we conducted a four-year experimental study, and conducted an experimental study on the pathogenesis, metastasis, and recurrence mechanism of tumor-bearing mice for three years, and an experimental study to explore how tumors cause host death. More than 1,000 tumor-bearing animals are used each year. In the model, nearly 6000 tumor-bearing animal models were made in 4 years. After the death of each mouse, the pathological anatomy of the liver, spleen, lung, thymus and kidney was performed. More than 20,000 slices were taken to explore whether it is possible. Tumor microvessels and microcirculation of 100 tumor-bearing mice were observed by microcirculation microscopy with microscopic pathogens.

Experimental results: Among the 200 kinds of Chinese herbal medicines screened by animal experiments in our laboratory, 48 kinds of selected and even excellent tumor cell proliferation were inhibited, and the tumor inhibition rate was above 75-90%. However, there are also some commonly used traditional Chinese medicines that are generally considered to have anti-cancer effects. After screening for animal tumors in vitro and in vivo, there is no anti-cancer effect, or the effect is very small. In this group, 152 kinds of anti-cancer effects were eliminated by animal experiments.

The 48 kinds of traditional Chinese medicines with good cancer suppression rate were selected by this experiment, and then the optimal combination of the two drugs was carried out, and the tumor-inhibiting rate experiment in the tumor-bearing body was repeated. Finally, the Chinese medicine with its own characteristics, XU ZE China$_{1-10}$ preparation (Z-C$_{1-10}$) are produced.

Z-C1 can significantly inhibit cancer cells, but does not affect normal cells; Z-C4 can promote thymic hyperplasia and increase immunity; Z-C8 can protect the marrow from hematopoiesis and protect bone marrow hematopoietic function.

5. clinical application, observation and verification

Clinical validation, based on the success of animal experiments, and then carried out clinical validation. That is to establish a tumor specialist clinic and a combination of Chinese and Western medicine for anti-cancer, anti-metastasis and recurrence research, retain the outpatient medical record, establish a regular follow-up observation system, and observe the long-term efficacy. From experimental research to clinical validation, new problems are discovered during the clinical validation process, and back to the laboratory for basic research, and new experimental results are applied to clinical validation. Thus, experimental-clinical-re-experiment-re-clinical, all experimental studies must be clinically verified, observed in a large number of patients for 3-5 years, and even clinical observations for 8-10 years, according to evidence-based medicine, with long-term follow-up And evaluable data, the evidence is clear that there is a good long-term efficacy, the standard of efficacy is: good quality of life, long life. Z-C immunomodulation anticancer traditional Chinese medicine preparation has been proved to be effective after being applied in a large number of patients with advanced cancer. Z-C immunomodulatory Chinese medicine can improve the quality of life of patients with advanced cancer, enhance immunity, increase the body's ability to fight cancer, enhance appetite, and significantly prolong survival.

Clinical application observation

1. Clinical data

The combination of Chinese and Western medicine combined with anti-cancer research, Hubei group, anti-cancer metastasis, recurrence research room and Shuguang oncology clinic, from November 1994 to November 2002, ZC immunomodulation of anti-cancer Chinese medicine combined with traditional Chinese medicine and western medicine for treatment III, IV or metastasis, there were 4698 cases of recurrent cancer, including 3051 males and 1647 females. The youngest is 11 years old, the largest is 86 years old, and the high age is 40 to 69 years old. **All patients were diagnosed by histopathological diagnosis or B-ultrasound, CT, MRI imaging. According to the International Anti-Cancer Alliance staging criteria, all cases were patients with intermediate stage III or higher stage, and this group of 1021 cases of liver cance**r, including 694 cases of primary liver cancer, 327 cases of metastatic liver cancer; 752 cases of lung cancer, including 699 cases of primary lung cancer There were 53 cases of metastatic lung cancer, 668 cases of gastric cancer, 624 cases of esophageal and cardiac cancer, 328 cases of rectal anal canal, 442 cases of colon cancer, 368 cases of breast cancer, 74 cases of pancreatic cancer, 30 cases of cholangiocarcinoma and 43 cases of retroperitoneal tumor. 38 cases of ovarian cancer, 9 cases of cervical cancer, 11 cases of brain tumor, 34 cases of thyroid cancer, 38 cases of nasopharyngeal carcinoma, 9 cases of melanoma, 27 cases of renal cell carcinoma, 48 cases of bladder cancer, 13 cases of white blood vessels, supraclavicular lymph node metastasis 47 cases, 35 cases of various sarcomas, 39 cases of other malignant tumors.

2. treatment effect

Symptoms improved, quality of life improved, and prolonged survival: In the 4277 middle- and late-stage cancer patients who were treated with Z-C immunomodulatory anti-cancer Chinese medicine for more than 3 months, the medical records were recorded in detail. Overall improvement in the quality of life of patients, see Table 1.

Table 1 4277 cases of efficacy observation to improve overall quality of life in patients with advanced cancer

Improvement	Spirit	Appetite	Physical strength	Enhance general situation	Wight increase	Sleep improvement	Improve activities and capacity restricted relief	Self-care Walking activity	Resume work as usual and Engaged in light body
Cases	4071	3986	2450	479	2938	1005	1038	3220	479
(%)	95.2	93.2	57.3	11.2	68.7	23.5	24.3	75.3	11.2

All the patients in the group were in the middle and advanced stage. After taking the medicine, they all had different degrees of symptom improvement, and the effective rate was 93.2%. In terms of improving the quality of life (according to the Kasper's scoring standard), the average score was 30 points before the drug administration, and after the drug was increased to an average of 80 points. The patients in this group had metastasis and dysfunction of different tissues and organs in the third stage or above.

The patients in this group had metastasis and dysfunction of different tissues and organs in stage III or above. The previous statistical data of such patients reported that the median survival time was about 6 months. The longest period of this group has reached 24 years, and the average survival time of other cases is more than 1 year. 1 case of primary hepatic lobe of hepatic lobe, recurrence of right liver after resection, treatment with ZC for 24 years; another case of ZC treatment for 20 years; 2 cases of hepatocellular carcinoma with multiple cancers in the liver, after taking ZC half year, during 2 times of CT scan the lesions completely disappeared and it has been stable for half a year. One case of double renal cell carcinoma, extensively transferred to the abdominal cavity after one side resection, was completely restored to work after taking Z-C medicine. In 3 cases of lung cancer the thoracotomy or the open chest exploration can not cut down and removed, the Z-C drug has been taken for 3 and a half years. Two cases of residual gastric cancer were treated with Z-C for 8 years. Three cases of rectal cancer had been treated with Z-C for 3 years. 1 case of breast cancer with metastasis of liver and ribs has been taken for 8 years. One case of recurrent bladder cancer after renal cell carcinoma disappeared for 9 and a half years after taking Z-C. **All of the above cases were inoperable, and could not be used in the middle and late stage of radiotherapy and chemotherapy. They were given Z-C medicine alone and were not treated with other drugs**.

So far, the patients still have come to the clinic every month to review and take medicine. After long-term medication, the condition is controlled in a stable state, so that the body and the tumor remain in a balanced state for a long time, and get better Survival with tumor, improved patient symptoms, improved quality of life, and the survival period is prolonged.

For 84 patients with solid mass and 56 patients with metastatic supraclavicular lymphadenopathy, Z-C system and external Z-C3 anti-cancer soft firming cream were obtained, which was better, see Table 2.

Table 2 Changes in 84 cases of solid masses and 56 cases of metastatic nodules after external application of Z-C cream

	Solid mass				cervical supraclavicular lymphadenopathy			
	disappear	Shrink 1/2	soft	No change	disappear	Shrink 1/2	soft	No change
Cases	12	28	32	12	12	22	14	8
(%)	14.2	33.3	38. 0	14.2	21.4	39.2	25.0	14.2
Total efficiency (%)	85.7				85.7			

6. Study on the mechanism of XZ-C immunoregulation of anticancer traditional Chinese medicine

Looking for anti-cancer and anti-metastatic new drugs in natural medicine (Chinese medicine) In our laboratory:

In the experimental work, our laboratory has carried out long-term and batch-by-batch experiments on the anti-tumor screening of tumor-bearing animals in 200 traditional Chinese medicines that are considered to be "anti-cancer Chinese medicines". It was found that only 48 of them had certain or even better inhibitory effects on the proliferation of tumor cells. After optimized combination, the tumor-inhibiting experiments in liver cancer, lung cancer, gastric cancer and other tumor-bearing animal models can form Z-C1-10 particles. Z-C1 can significantly inhibit cancer cells, but does not affect normal cells. Z-C4 can protect the chest. Ascending and exempting, improving immune function, Z-C8 can protect the marrow and raise blood. ZC immunoregulatory Chinese medicine can improve the quality of life of patients with advanced cancer, increase immunity, enhance physical fitness, increase appetite and prolong survival.

With the deepening of research on traditional Chinese medicine, many traditional Chinese medicines are known to regulate the production and biological activities of cytokines and other immune molecules. This is of great significance for elucidating the immunological mechanism of Z-C immunomodulation of anticancer Chinese medicine at the molecular level.

(1) **XZ-C anti-cancer Chinese medicine can protect immune organs and increase the weight of thymus and spleen**
(2) **Effects of Z-C anticancer Chinese medicine on proliferation, differentiation and hematopoietic function of bone marrow cells**
(3) **Z-C anticancer Chinese medicine has enhanced T cell immune function**

7. Characteristics of traditional Chinese medicine immunopharmacology

Compared with Western medicine immunopharmacology, traditional Chinese medicine immunopharmacology has its own characteristics or advantages, and each has its own shortcomings. The advantages of traditional Chinese medicine immunology are as follows:

First of all, long-term clinical experience has accumulated a large number of prescriptions to regulate the body's immune function, especially the tonics or beneficial Chinese medicines generally have the effect of regulating immune activity.

Traditional Chinese medicine is rich in sources. In recent years, research has increasingly proved that traditional Chinese medicine is an effective medicine for long-term clinical treatment. After extraction, it can obtain obvious pharmacological effects (including immunomodulatory effects), and the research process saves people time and has high efficiency.

Secondly, traditional Chinese medicines, whether single-agent or prescription, contain multiple active ingredients, unlike Western medicine (synthetic drugs), which are single-structured substances. The role of traditional Chinese medicine is multifaceted. In addition to regulating immune function, it has a certain effect on the whole functional system and organs. And these roles are connected and combined.

The role of traditional Chinese medicine in regulating immune function is generally tonics or supporting the good things or beneficial, that is, within the normal adjustment range, **two-way regulation is the main feature**. The tonic drug can be called immunomodulatory drugs, causing a non-specific immune response.

Replenishment class of traditional Chinese medicine or tonics or supporting the body strength has the role of regulating the body's immune function. Under the general experimental conditions, the correlation between dose and benefit is presented, especially in normal healthy animal experiments. When the animal is at a low level of immune activity (such as dethymus, aging animals or chemotherapy drugs cyclophosphamide inhibition and tumor animals), the tonic drugs improve the body's immunity is more significant.

Immunopharmacology is an interdisciplinary subject formed by the combination of immunology and pharmacology. Traditional Chinese medicine immunopharmacology plays a special important role in immunopharmacology in China. Traditional Chinese medicine immunopharmacology can be understood as a new discipline in the grafting of traditional Chinese medicine and modern immunopharmacology.

As early as the 1970s, Professor Zhou Jin had been calling for the establishment of pharmacology in the integration of Chinese and Western medicine in China, and clearly proposed to study and clarify the pharmacological effects of traditional Chinese medicine from the theory of traditional Chinese medicine.

TCM theory has its obvious overall view, emphasizing the balance of the body and maintaining balance when the internal and external environment changes. Losing balance and coordination, the body will have a medical certificate.

Modern medicine also emphasizes the stability of the internal environment. The regulatory factors for the stability of the internal environment are the three systems of nerve, endocrine and immunity. These are self-contained systems that independently exert their respective regulatory roles, while at the same time interacting with each other and interacting with each other to achieve the goal of maintaining a relatively stable internal environment. "Nerve, endocrine, immune, regulatory networks" (NIM network) is currently a research hotspot in immunopharmacology. Professor Zhou Jin developed the NIM idea through a lot of research work, and believed that the "NIM" concept has broad practical significance, is in line with the laws of life science, and coincides with the overall ideology of traditional Chinese medicine. Extensive and in-depth study of the role of traditional Chinese medicine in the NIM network can greatly develop the basic theories of Chinese medicine, so that Chinese medicine can go global faster.

8. XZ-C immunomodulation anticancer Chinese medicine is the result of the modernization of traditional Chinese medicine

XZ-C immunomodulation anticancer traditional Chinese medicine is not an empirical method, nor is it an old Chinese medicine practitioner. It is the scientific research achievement of the combination of Chinese and Western medicine and the modernization of traditional Chinese medicine. It is a modern medical method, using experimental tumor research methods and modern pharmacology and medicine. Combining the effects of research methods, after 7 years of more than 4 000 cancer-bearing animal models, 200 commonly used anti-cancer Chinese herbal medicines were screened in batches for animal experiments, and the tumor inhibition rate in vitro and in tumor-bearing animals was screened and screened. There are 48 kinds of traditional Chinese medicines with anti-cancer effects; then make these 48 kinds of natural medicines into XZ-C1-10, and according to respiratory system, digestive system, urinary system, gynecology, endocrine system to manufacture cancer-bearing animal models of various systems of liver cancer, gastric cancer, colon cancer, breast cancer, bladder cancer, and lung cancer, then carrying out pharmacodynamic experiments and toxicological experiments in tumor-bearing animals. It is made into XZ-C1, XZ-C2, XZ-C3, XZ-C4, XZ-C5, XZ-C6, XZ-C7, XZ-C8 and other series of immunomodulatory anticancer Chinese medicines.

The material basis for the traditional prescription to exert its unique therapeutic effect is the chemical composition, the change of the quality and quantity of the chemical composition, which directly affects the clinical efficacy of the prescription. Therefore, only by studying the changes in the quality and quantity of chemical components in the prescriptions, to find out the main active ingredients of the preparations, and to explore the mysteries of their unique effects from the perspective of molecular immunology, can the research of traditional prescriptions take a new step.

XZ-C immunomodulation Chinese medicine preparation is an innovation and reform of traditional Chinese medicine preparation. It is not a mixed decoction compound liquid, but a particle concentrate or powder for each flavor medicine. The raw medicine of each flavor remains the original ingredient in each medicine. The role, molecular weight, structural formula is unchanged, made by modern scientific methods, not compound, keep the original ingredients and functions of each flavor unchanged, easy to evaluate, affirm the role and efficacy of the drug.

9. In the field of cancer research, traditional Chinese medicine is an advantage of China. In "How to improve immunity?", Chinese herbal medicine has an extremely important advantage.

Many of Chinese herbal medicines are immune enhancers, biological response modifiers, and tonics, many of which can strengthen the body's immunity and anti-cancer power. The two world diseases that currently threaten human life are cancer and AIDS. The former is immunocompromised and the latter is immunodeficient. At present, scientists all over the world agree that tumor formation is summarized into three processes: the first step is that carcinogenic factors act on the body and interfere with cell metabolism; the second step is to disrupt the genetic information in the nucleus and cause cell cancer; the third step is that the cancer cells escape the body. The immune alert defense system, the body's immune defense ability is an internal cause, and the external cause works through internal factors. Cancer cells must be able to escape the monitoring system of the body's alarm system, break through the body's immune defense line, then develop into a tumor. Therefore, trying to improve the body's immunity is the key measure to prevent cancer and cancer. How to improve immunity? Chinese herbal medicine is an extremely important advantage. There are many kinds of immune Chinese herbal medicine preparations with rich drug sources. It should be used as an important anti-cancer, anti-AIDS resource, tissue research and development.

The prevention and treatment of malignant tumors are all underway in the world. All countries have concentrated a large number of experts and scholars with experimental research ability and clinical practice experience to try to overcome cancer.

We should give full play to China's advantages in the areas where our country has advantages and catch up with the international advanced level.

In the field of cancer research, traditional Chinese medicine is an advantage of China. To play the role of this advantage in the field of cancer research, to explore and develop anti-cancer, anti-cancer herbal medicines, to play this advantage, should be a strategic vision of international significance.

On the road of human conquest of cancer, research, discovery, and development of effective and repeatable new anti-cancer and anti-cancer Chinese herbal preparations can certainly make a difference, and can be tapped into effective treasures. It must be carried out the strict, objective, factual, and scientifically repeated research using rigorous scientific methods and modern experimental surgical methods. All experimental research must pass strict clinical verification. In a large number of patients, the evidence is clear and indeed has good curative effect. The standard of curative effect is good quality of life and prolonged survival.

III. XZ-C's Scientific research, scientific thinking, academic thinking, scientific dedication or contribution is to take 'Conquer Cancer 'as a research direction

Contents

Exploring the etiology, pathogenesis and pathophysiology of cancer
An effective way to find regulation

- Experimental research on the production of cancer animal models
- Exploring the experimental study of the relationship between tumors and immune organs, looking for ways to control immune

- Exploring experimental studies to curb thymic atrophy in tumor progression and to find immune reconstruction methods
- Find medicines that inhibit tumor angiogenesis from natural medicines

Thymus atrophy and low immune function are one of the causes and pathogenesis of cancer

- New findings in experimental research on the etiology, pathogenesis and pathophysiology of cancer
- Explore ways to curb tumor progression, progressive atrophy of the thymus, and immune reconstitution

Theoretical basis and experimental basis of XZ-C protection of 'Thymus and incrase of immune function' immunomodulatory therapy

- Animal experiment enlightenment
- Protect, regulate, and activate the anti-cancer immune system in the human body
- Overview of research on anti-cancer Chinese medicines
- XZ-C immunoregulation of traditional Chinese medicines
- XZ-C immunomodulation Chinese medicine clinical application principles and scope of application

Experimental observation of tumor on thymus and spleen of immune organs

- Animal experiment research

Group of experimental animals
experimental method
Experimental result

- After vaccination of cancer cells, the thymus shows progressive atrophy throughout the course of the disease, cell proliferation is blocked, and the thymus is extremely atrophied in the late stage of the tumor.
- The thymus of the tumor-bearing mice showed a regular change. After the 7th day of inoculation of the cancer cells, it showed acute progressive atrophy, cell proliferation was blocked, and the thymus was extremely atrophied in the late stage, and the immune function was also decreased or even lost.
- The cellular immune function of the body is increasingly inhibited as the tumor progresses, causing immune dysfunction and tumor growth.

- Protect the thymus to improve immunity, protect bone marrow, enhance hematopoietic function, improve immunity and regulation, comprehensively improve the quality of life of patients with advanced cancer, and improve treatment effect
- XZ-C immunomodulation anticancer Chinese medicine is the result of the modernization of traditional Chinese medicine.

First, the theoretical system of XZ-C immunomodulation and cancer treatment has been formed. Over the past 60 years, a new road to overcome cancer has been taken out. It is undergoing clinical application and observation verification.

1. New findings in anti-cancer and anti-cancer metastasis research
2. Experimental observation of the effect of tumor on immune thymus
3. Morphology and location of the thymus
4. the structure of the thymus, the function of the thymus
5. the body's immune function
6. thymus immune regulation function, NIM theory
7. thymus exocrine function
8. Effect of chemical drugs on immune function of the body
9. the naming and function of thymus hormone
10. immune regulation, immune promoter
11. Research progress on anticancer immune pharmacology of traditional Chinese medicine polysaccharides
12. Characteristics of traditional Chinese medicine immunopharmacology
13. Discovered from experimental tumor research
14. Study on the mechanism of XZ-C immunoregulation of anticancer Chinese medicine
15. XZ-C anti-cancer Chinese medicine induces cytokines
16. Experimental and clinical efficacy of XZ-C immunomodulation anticancer Chinese medicine
17. XZ-C immunomodulation anticancer Chinese medicine is the result of the modernization of traditional Chinese medicine

Second, find the way

1. Exploring the mechanisms of cancer pathogenesis, invasion and recurrence and metastasis, and conducting experimental research on effective measures to control invasion, recurrence and metastasis

2. looking for new anti-cancer, anti-metastatic, anti-recurrence new drug experiments from natural drugs
3. How to find new ways to regulate immune therapy
4. clinical verification work
5. Study on the mechanism of XZ-C immunoregulation of anticancer traditional Chinese medicine
6. XZ-C immunomodulation anticancer Chinese medicine is the result of modernization of traditional Chinese medicine
7. take XZ-C immune regulation, molecular level, Western medicine combined with the road to overcome cancer

A. The First Article

"Theoretical basis and experimental basis of immune regulation and treatment of cancer"

The new findings in animal experiment research

We have been conducting a full-scale clinical research work in the laboratory for 4 years. It is a clinical basic research. The topic of the research project is a clinically-provided problem, in order to explain these clinical problems or solve these clinical problems through experimental research.

From the results of a series of animal experiments exploring the etiology, pathogenesis and pathophysiology of cancer, we have revealed that thymus atrophy leads to low immunity, and then immune surveillance declines, eventually developing into immune escape, which may be one of the key causes of cancer etiology and pathogenesis. It is a new development of 21st century oncology theory, which provides direction and basis for cancer therapeutics in the 21st century, and provides theoretical basis and experimental basis for cancer immune regulation treatment. This innovative discovery has not been mentioned in textbooks and literature at home and abroad. It is the first time in the world, and it is an original paper and an international initiative.

XZ-C is the scientific research, scientific thinking, and scientific dedication and achievement based on "conquer cancer" as the research direction, which the brief introduction is:

Chapter I

The New Discovery of the Follow-up Results

This is a new series of findings from clinical follow-up, from the clinical problems, problems found, the following series of experimental basic research and clinical validation observations.

cause:

(1) Why do I study cancer? I am a clinical surgeon, why do you study cancer? This is due to the results of a petition to a group of cancer patients after surgery.

In 1985, I conducted a petition with more than 3,000 patients who underwent radical surgery for various cancers outside the chest (all according to the operating room registration list). It was found that most patients relapsed and metastasized 2 to 3 years after surgery. This made me realize that although the operation is successful, the long-term efficacy is not satisfactory. Postoperative recurrence and metastasis are the key factors affecting the long-term efficacy of the operation. It also reminds us that prevention and treatment of postoperative recurrence and metastasis is the key to prolonging postoperative survival. Therefore, clinical basic research must be carried out. Without breakthroughs in basic research, clinical efficacy is difficult to improve, so we established the Institute of Experimental Surgery and conducted a series of experimental research and clinical validation work.

(2) From the results of follow-up, it was found that:

1. postoperative recurrence and metastasis are the key factors affecting the long-term efficacy of surgery;
2. prompt clinicians must pay attention to and study the prevention and treatment of postoperative recurrence and metastasis, in order to improve the long-term effect of surgery

(3) Through large-scale follow-up, I found an important issue: postoperative recurrence and metastasis are the key factors affecting the long-term efficacy of surgery. Therefore, we also raised an important issue: Studying the method of preventing and treating postoperative recurrence and metastasis of cancer is the key to improving the long-term efficacy of

surgery, which is the key to improve the postoperative survival of patients. Therefore, clinical basic research to prevent cancer recurrence and metastasis must be carried out. Without breakthroughs in basic research, clinical efficacy is difficult to improve. So we established an experimental surgery laboratory, conducted experimental tumor research, performed cancer cell transplantation, established a tumor animal model, and carried out a series of experimental tumor research: exploring cancer recurrence, metastasis mechanism and regularity; exploring tumors and immune and immune organs and The relationship between immune organs and tumors; to explore ways to suppress progressive atrophy of immune organs and to re-immunize tumors; to find effective measures to regulate invasion, recurrence and metastasis of cancer; to consider the commonly used anti-cancer Chinese herbal medicines in 200 literatures Experimental screening of tumor suppressor rate in cancer-bearing solid tumors; experimental research on new drugs against cancer, anti-metastasis and anti-recurrence from natural drugs. Using modern science and technology, in-depth study of the discovery of anti-cancer and anti-cancer Chinese herbal medicine. In the traditional anti-cancer Chinese herbal medicine, a strict, scientific and repeated tumor-bearing animal model was screened in vivo, and no stable effect was eliminated. 48 kinds of Z-C immunoregulatory and traditional Chinese medicines with good curative effect were screened out. It has been applied to clinical practice on the basis of the success of animal experiments. After 34 years of clinical trials of a large number of clinical cases, the curative effect is remarkable.

Chapter II

The New Discovery of the Animal Experimental Research

1. The new discovery summary from the cancer experimental study of anti-cancer and anti-metastasis and anti-recurrence

(1) In our laboratory, the thymus (Thymus, TH) (30 mice) was excised from mice, and a tumor-bearing animal model can be made. The injection of immunosuppressive drugs can also contribute to the establishment of a cancer-bearing animal model. The conclusion of the study proves that the occurrence and development of cancer have obvious relationship with the thymus and its function of the host immune organs.

(2) Whether it is immune first and then easy to get cancer, or cancer first and then low immunity, the experimental results are: first, there is low immunity and then the occurrence and development of cancer, if no immune function declines, it is not easy to vaccinate successfully. **The results of this experiment suggest that improving and maintaining good immune function is one of the important measures to prevent cancer.**

(3) When we studied the relationship between metastasis and immunity of cancer, we established 60 animal models of liver metastases, and divided them into group A and group B with immunosuppressive drugs, and group B did not. RESULTS: The number of intrahepatic metastases in group A was significantly higher than that in group B. The results of this experiment suggest:

Metastasis is associated with immunity, low immune function or the use of immunosuppressive drugs may promote tumor metastasis.

(4) When we explored the effect of tumor on the immune organs of the body, we found that as the cancer progresses, the thymus is progressively atrophied (600 mice bearing cancer model mice), and the host thymus presented acute progressive atrophy after inoculation of cancer cells.

(5) It was also found through experiments that some of the experimental mice did not vaccinate successfully, or the tumor grew small, the thymus did not shrink significantly.

In order to understand the relationship between tumor and thymus atrophy, we removed tumor in a group of experimental mice when the transplanted solid tumor grew to the size of the thumb. After 1 month, the thymus was found to have no progressive atrophy. Therefore, we speculate that a solid tumor may produce a factor that is not known to inhibit the thymus, which needs further study.

(6)   The above experimental results prove that the progression of the tumor can cause progressive atrophy of the thymus. Then, can we adopt some methods to prevent the host thymus from shrinking? Therefore, we further designed and tried to find ways or drugs to prevent thymus atrophy in tumor-bearing mice through animal experiments. Therefore, we used this immune organ cell transplantation to restore the experimental function of the immune organ.

We are investigating the atrophy of the thymus gland in suppressing tumor progression, looking for ways to restore the function of the thymus and reconstituting the immune system. The mice were transplanted with fetal liver, fetal spleen and fetal thymus cells, and the immune function of the immune system was re-established. Results: S, T, L three groups of cells (200 rats), the recent complete tumor regression rate was 40%, the long-term tumor complete regression rate was 46.67%, the tumor completely disappeared long-term survival.

What causes the thymus to shrink?

It may be that the tumor produces an immunosuppressive factor that inhibits the thymus.

XZ-C believes that it can be temporarily called "cancer inhibiting Thymus (TH) factor", which needs further experimental research.

In order to explore the etiology, pathogenesis and pathophysiology of cancer, we conducted a series of animal experiments, **from the results of experimental research to analyze and think, so that we can obtain new discoveries, new thinking, new enlightenment: one of the causes of cancer It may be atrophy of the thymus, impaired thymus function, and low immune function. Therefore, Professor Xu Ze proposed one of the causes and pathogenesis of cancer at international conferences, which may be thymus atrophy, impaired central immune organ function, low immune function, decreased immune surveillance ability and immune escape. But what is the cause of the host's thymus atrophy? After repeated thinking and speculation, it may be because a factor produced by solid tumors inhibits the thymus, but this needs further experimental research, we can temporarily call it "cancer Thymus suppressive factor".**

Looking back on the research history of cancer in the past 100 years, the research on the etiology, pathophysiology and pathogenesis of cancer is still rare. In the past 100 years, people have made efforts in clinical research and pathological research of cancer in the fields of surgery, radiotherapy and chemotherapy. Laboratory basic research and clinical basic research such as mutation, cloning, proliferation, metastasis, and planting regularity, such as invasion, metastasis, tumor thrombus, immunity, and endocrine, are relatively rare. Many large hospitals have not established laboratories for clinical basic research. **Reviewing and reflecting on the experience and lessons of the author's clinical surgery for more than 60 years, it is clear that without clinical breakthroughs, clinical efficacy is difficult to improve.**

From the experimental tumor research findings In order to explore the cause, pathogenesis, invasion and metastasis mechanism of cancer, and find effective measures for regulation, intervention, invasion, recurrence and metastasis, the author and colleagues conducted a full four-year experimental tumor research work.

(1) Experiment 1: Excision of mouse thymus (Thymus, TH) to produce a tumor-bearing animal model, injection of immunosuppressive drugs contribute to the establishment of a cancer-bearing animal model. The research conclusions show that the occurrence and development of cancer have a significant correlation with the thymus and function of the host immune organs.

(2) Experiment 2: Whether it is immune first and then easy to get cancer, or cancer first and then low immunity, the experimental results confirmed that the first immune system is low and then easy to have cancer, the development, if no immune function decline, it is not easy to vaccinate success. The experimental results suggest that improving and maintaining good immune function, and protecting the central immune organ thymus is one of the important measures to prevent cancer.

(3) Experiment 3: In the study of the relationship between cancer metastasis and immunity, an animal model of liver metastasis was established and divided into two groups, A and B groups. Group A used immunosuppressive drugs, and group B did not. Results The number of intrahepatic metastases in group A was significantly higher than that in group B. The experimental results suggest that metastasis is associated with immunity, low immune function or the use of immunosuppressive drugs can promote tumor metastasis.

(4) Experiment 4: When investigating the effect of tumor on immune organs, it was found that with the progress of cancer, the thymus showed progressive atrophy, and the host thymus was acute progressive atrophy after inoculation of cancer cells, and cell proliferation was blocked. The volume is significantly reduced. The experimental results suggest that the tumor may inhibit the thymus and cause the immune organs to shrink.

(5) Experiment 5: It was found in the experiment that some of the experimental mice did not have a successful vaccination or the tumor grew very small, and the thymus did not significantly shrink. To understand the relationship between tumor and thymus atrophy, a group of experimental mice transplanted solid tumors were resected when they reached the size of the thumb. After 1 month of dissection, it was found that the thymus did not undergo progressive atrophy. **Therefore, we speculate that a solid tumor may produce a factor that is not yet known to inhibit the thymus, which needs further study**.

It is generally believed that the immune function of the body affects the occurrence, development and prognosis of the tumor, and the tumor also has an inhibitory effect on the immune state of the body. The two are causal and intricate.

Why does the host's thymus show acute progressive atrophy after inoculation of cancer cells, cell proliferation is blocked, and the volume is significantly reduced? It suggests that the tumor may have an inhibitory effect, causing the immune organs to shrink. But what factors or factors cause thymus atrophy, Professor Xu Ze believes that the tumor may produce immunosuppressive factors causing thymus atrophy, XZ-C believes that it may be temporarily called "Thymus (TH) factor."

About the immunosuppressive effects of tumors:

The above experiment explored the effect of tumor on the immune organs of the body. It was found that with the progress of cancer, the thymus showed progressive atrophy. The host thymus was acutely progressively atrophied after inoculation of cancer cells, cell proliferation was blocked, and the volume was significantly reduced.

During the experiment, many changes were observed in the thymus of the immune organs of the tumor-bearing mice. It seems that there was a certain regularity in the cost of living. The host thymus was acutely progressively atrophied after inoculation of cancer cells. The thymus does not shrink. When the solid tumor inoculated into the mouse is resected to the size of the thumb, the thymus does not shrink again.

The above clarifies that the relationship between inoculated cancer cells and host thymus atrophy has a certain regularity, and there is a certain correlation. Why is the acute progressive atrophy of the host thymus after successful cancer cell inoculation?

The results suggest that the tumor may inhibit the thymus causing atrophy of the immune organs, but what factors or factors cause the thymus atrophy, therefore, we speculate that the solid tumor may produce a factor that is not yet known to inhibit the thymus Professor Xu Ze believes that it can be temporarily called **"cancer Thymus suppressor factor"** and needs further experimental research.

XZ-C believes that **"cancer inhibiting Thymus factor"** may be a tumor-derived immunosuppressive factor that induces the production of immunosuppressive T cells (TS cells), which have immunosuppressive effects.

Immunosuppressive effects of tumors: The occurrence, development, metastasis and recurrence of cancer are closely related to immune system hypoplasia and immune dysfunction.

The body's immune system dysfunction, immune function is prone to malignant tumors: such as animal resection of thymus, chemotherapy drugs, radiation, adrenocortical hormones, etc. can inhibit the body's immune status, as well as long-term use of immunosuppressive drugs or long-term chemotherapy, The incidence of tumors was high.

Malignant tumors **invade the** immune organs and cause immune function decline or inhibition. They can also release immunosuppressive factors, reduce host immunity or induce inhibitory cell growth in the body. The immune function of patients with metaphase malignant tumors is generally low, but when the tumor is surgically removed, the disease is relieved. After that, the immune function will have different degrees of recovery. This may indicate that the tumor has immunosuppressive effects. Therefore, it is suggested that clinical cancer treatment should pay attention to immune regulation treatment.

Tumor immunosuppression has the following aspects:

1. Inhibitory cells: mostly inhibitory T cells (TS fine) and inhibitory macrophages. TS cells of tumor-bearing mice can release specific inhibitory factors in vitro, directly acting on effector cells and inhibiting CTL cells.
2. Production of immunosuppressive factors:

Tumor-derived immunosuppressive factor: A tumor-derived suppressor factor (TDSF) was found to induce TS cell production from mouse fibrosarcoma.

The above experimental studies suggest that one of the causes of cancer and the pathogenesis may be thymus atrophy, thymocyte proliferation is blocked, thymus function is impaired, immune function is low, and the immune escape of malignant cells is caused.

Since the thymus develops progressive atrophy as the tumor progresses, how do you intervene to prevent it from shrinking? Animal experimental studies were conducted to find ways or drugs to prevent thymic atrophy in tumor-bearing mice.

New findings from the above experiments suggest that thymus atrophy and low immune function are one of the causes and pathogenesis of cancer, so we should look for methods, techniques, and drugs to prevent thymic atrophy and prevent immune dysfunction.

To prevent thymic atrophy, you should try to stop the "cancer suppressor factor."

To prevent immune deficiencies, you should try to improve the body's immune function, or immune regulation, or immune reconstitution.

<u>**In summary, the treatment of cancer must be treated with immunomodulation**</u>.

Current methods for immunomodulation or immune reconstitution: **one is to transplant immune cells from biological cells for immune reconstitution; one is to find the immune regulate and control chinese medicine with activating cytokines, enhancing immune surveillance, thereby inhibiting tumors and preventing immunity from thymic atrophy from natural medicines such as Chinese herbal medicines.**

In 1986, at the satellite conference of the International Microcirculation Conference, the author was inspired to find ways to improve microcirculation drugs from natural medicines, and **<u>then shift adoptive immunization from biological cell transplantation for reconstitute the immune system into seeking for activating cytokines from natural medicines such as Chinese herbal medicines, enhance immune surveillance, thereby inhibiting tumors and preventing thymus atrophy</u>**. All drugs must pass animal experiments and clinical validation. So in the study of cancer-bearing animal models, after 3 years, more than 200 kinds of traditional Chinese medicines were sterilized and screened from natural medicines, and finally, anti-cancer immune regulation Chinese medicines with good anti-tumor effects were screened out. After clinical screening and clinical verification, it is further filtered from Chinese medicine immunology and concentrated into XZ-C$_{1-10}$ anti-cancer immune regulation Chinese medicine, which can promote thymic hyperplasia, prevent thymus atrophy, enhance immune function and protect bone marrow. Promote T lymphocyte function and cytokines, and have a high tumor inhibition rate, only inhibit cancer cells without affecting normal cells, and can be taken orally for a long time. Because cancer is a chronic disease, the division, proliferation, and cloning of cancer cells are long-term, continuous, and progressive, so it is advisable to use non-toxic, orally-administered sustained-release drugs for long-term use.

Chinese herbal medicine for treating cancer is to treat the cause and pathogenesis from the overall perspective of human beings, not to kill cancer cells, but also to improve the body's autoimmune function, thereby enhancing the body's anti-cancer ability, so it can make some refractory and extensive transfer. The cancer is controlled, prolonging the life of cancer patients, alleviating the suffering of patients, and opening up a new path for cancer treatment to combine cancer with Chinese and Western medicine.

A series of experimental studies on the etiology, pathogenesis, and pathophysiology of cancer have revealed that thymus atrophy leads to low immune function, and then immune surveillance declines, eventually developing into immune escape, which may be one of the key causes of cancer etiology and pathogenesis. It is a new development of 21st century oncology theory, which provides direction and basis for cancer therapeutics in the 21st century, and provides theoretical basis and experimental basis for cancer immune regulation treatment. This innovative discovery has not been mentioned in textbooks and literature at home and abroad. It is the first time in the world, and it is an original paper and an international initiative.

2. The Animal Experimental Research (1)

Exploring the experimental study of the etiology, pathogenesis and pathophysiology of cancer, and finding an effective method for regulation and control

In 1985, the author conducted a petition to more than 3,000 patients who had undergone various postoperative chest cancer operations. The results of follow-up showed that the vast majority of patients relapsed and metastasized from 2 to 3 years after surgery; some even relapsed and died within a few months after surgery. It is thought that the operation is successful, the long-term treatment is unsatisfactory, or it fails. The patient underwent a major operation and only lived for one or two years or 2-3 years. Obviously this is not a requirement for the patient to treat the disease. And the purpose is not what the doctor wants to see. Usually we read the literature only pay attention to the 5-year survival rate and not pay attention to the 5-year mortality rate, such as a group of gastric cancer 5 years postoperative survival rate of 20%, in turn, its 5-year mortality rate is 80%, such a high postoperative The 5-year mortality rate shocked patients and their families. A large number of follow-up results found an important problem: **postoperative**

recurrence and metastasis are the key factors affecting the long-term efficacy of surgery. At the same time, an important issue has been raised: the study of methods and measures for prevention and treatment of postoperative recurrence and metastasis is the key to determining the long-term efficacy of surgery, which is the key to improving the postoperative survival of patients.

The current recurrence and metastasis rate is still quite high, of course, it is related to many factors such as tumor stage, grading, differentiation and immune function of the body. There are still many cases of recurrence and metastasis in the outpatient clinic. In one week, the author saw 40 cases in the clinic. The patient, that is, 15 patients who had recurrence after surgery, roughly analyzed these cases and relapsed several months after surgery. It can be seen that postoperative recurrence and metastasis must be started from the surgery. Because cancer resection is prone to residue, tumor cells are prone to planting and dissemination, and once there is residual or disseminated, recurrence and metastasis are very likely to occur, and the consequences are often unimaginable. Therefore, the implementation of tumor surgery must follow the basic principles of surgical surgery. The principle of performing tumor-free techniques for tumor surgery must be as strict or even more stringent as the surgeon's principles of aseptic technique. **The implementation of the principle of no-tumor technology has two main purposes: one is to prevent dissemination, and the other is to prevent planting.**

The key to determining the long-term outcome of surgery is recurrence and metastasis. In the 20th century, surgeons have achieved brilliant achievements in cancer surgical resection techniques. The task of surgeons in the 21st century should be to prevent postoperative recurrence and metastasis in order to improve the long-term efficacy of surgical treatment.

If there is no breakthrough in basic research, the clinical efficacy is difficult to improve. If the problem of recurrence and metastasis after surgery is studied and solved, the surgical treatment of solid tumors will achieve even more brilliant achievements.

Therefore, in 1985, the author established a laboratory of experimental surgery in clinical surgery, and carried out research on experimental tumors. First, he explored the manufacture of experimental tumor models and began to move from clinical to basic experimental research.

To explore the etiology, pathogenesis and metastasis mechanism of cancer, and **to explore the prevention and treatment methods from multiple links of cancer cell metastasis**. In the past seven years, the research projects have been clinical issues, aiming to explain or solve some clinical problems through experimental research.

Through 7 years of animal experiment research, we carried out a layer-by-step and step-by-step study on the basic problems, and then completed the following experimental research work.

I. Experimental study on the manufacture of animal models of cancer

Why do people get cancer? What state of the body will get cancer? Why do people get cancer in the same environment and under the same conditions? Is it due to internal or external causes, or internal and external causes? To this end, we should make a model of tumor-bearing animals.

(1) Conducting experimental research on tumors to produce a cancer-bearing animal model

At that time, the author was the director of clinical surgery and the director of the experimental surgery research department of the Affiliated Hospital of Hubei University of Traditional Chinese Medicine. It facilitated the coordination and coordination of the work of clinical wards and animal laboratories, and removed the specimens of sterile tumors on the clinical operating table. After warm ischemia 0. 5h, then transplanted on experimental animals, and more than 100 times (400 animals) were unsuccessful. Subsequent re-transplantation of the cancer cells in mice with resected thymus was successful (210 animals), and some were injected with cortisone, which reduced the immunity of the mice, was also successfully transplanted. After 5 days of thymusectomy, in 5-6d a large nodule of soybeans can grow, at the 10-21d it grew into a large tumor of thumb size. Transplanted cancer can survive for 3-4 weeks, but cannot be pass next generation.

1. Through this study, it was found that excision of the thymus can produce a model of a cancer-bearing animal, and injection of cortisone can also help to produce a cancer-bearing animal model.

2. The research conclusions show that the occurrence and development of cancer is related to the host's immunity, and it has a very obvious relationship with the immune organs and immune organs.

3. The results of this study confirmed that the immune system thymus (Thymus, Th) and immune function have a very definite relationship with the occurrence and development of cancer. If the host Th is removed, it may be a model of a cancer-bearing animal. Without resection, it cannot cause cancer. In animal models, injection of an immunosuppressive drug to reduce host immunity can help to create a model of a cancer-bearing animal. Without the injection of a reduced immunological drug, a cancer-bearing animal model cannot be produced. This result indicates that immune organs and immunity are negatively correlated with cancer cell transplantation, implantation and growth into solid cancer. If the immune defect or immune is reduced, the transplant can grow into a tumor and not be swallowed by the host's immune cell recognition.

(2) Whether it is decreasing immune first, then cancer occurrence, or is it cancer occurrence first, then immune decreasing?

A total of 320 Kunming mice were divided into group A, group B, group C and group D, with n=80 in each group. The thymectomy and transplantation method were the same as before. Group A was the first to remove the thymus, and 5 days after inoculation of cancer cells 10^6. Group B was injected with cortisone first, and then cancer cells were inoculated after 7 days; group C was first inoculated with cancer cells, and thymus was removed after l0d; group D was first inoculated with tumor cells, and cortisone was injected after l0d. As a result, both groups A and B were successfully vaccinated and grew small tumors, in group C and group D only 18 of them had mung bean tumors after 14 days. **The results of this experiment suggest that the**

immune function of the host is reduced first, or the thymus of the immune organ is defective to grow the tumor. If the host immune function is good, it is not easy to grow a tumor, and it can be concluded that the immune function is low and then the cancer develops. If the immune function is not reduced first, it is not easy to vaccinate successfully. This study suggests that improving and maintaining good immune function and protecting well-functioning immune organs is an important measure to prevent cancer.

(3) Modeling experiment of cancer metastasis model

Regarding cancer cell transplantation research, in 1985, the author conducted a solid cancer transplantation model by transplanting dozens of human cancer cells into the thymus-free mice in the experimental surgery laboratory. Later, a cancer metastasis model was performed to simulate lymphatic metastasis. We transplanted 10^6/mI, 0.2 ml of H22 cell suspension subcutaneously on the inside of 60 mouse paw pads. After 7-8d, the inside of the paw pad grew a large tumor of broad bean. The entire foot was swollen and entrapped.

After 16 days, 8 mice found a right inguinal lymph node enlargement **and established a lymphatic metastasis model.** After that, **the author simulated blood transfer**, and injected H22 cell suspension 106 / ml, 0.4 m1 into the human vein intravenously, obtained more lung metastasis, causing tumor growth in the lung. Subsequently, an experimental animal model of liver metastasis was established. 80 Kunming mice were divided into groups A and B, 40 in each group.

Group A was first injected with cortisone for 7 days, and was anesthetized by intraperitoneal injection of I% pentobarbital sodium 75 mg/kg. Then, the left middle abdomen was made into a 0.5 cm incision, exposed to the spleen, and the live H_{22} liver cancer ascites 10 ul. Subcutaneous injection, local compression for 3-5min, to prevent cancer cells from spilling into the peritoneal spleen and injecting cancer cells into the lymph and blood. After the animals were reared for 11 days, the neck was broken and the liver was taken for colony colony counting. As a result, there were liver cancer metastasis in the liver of group A. B. The number of intrahepatic metastases was different. The number of group A was significantly higher than that of group B, mostly 3-5 or more, and the diameter was about 1 mm. The majority of group B is 1 to 3 cancer lesions.

The experimental results suggest that

Metastasis is associated with clear immunity, low immune function, or the use of drugs that inhibit immunity, which can promote tumor metastasis.

II, to explore the experimental study of the relationship between tumors and immune organs, seeking ways of immune regulation and control

As the laboratory explored the establishment of experimental cancer-bearing animal models, it was found that resection of the thymus, reduction of immunity or immunodeficiency can establish an animal model of cancer transplantation, then the thymus is definitely associated with the growth of cancer, and the thymus is the center of Immune organs, the spleen is the largest peripheral immune organ, what is the relationship between the spleen and the tumor? In order to further study and study the relationship between immune organs and tumorigenesis and development, the author conducted an experimental study on the next topic.

(1)   Experimental study on the effect of **spleen** on tumor growth

In view of the fact that the spleen is a peripheral immune organ with important immune function, it plays an important role in anti-tumor immunity. **In order to investigate the effect of spleen on tumor growth and its changes, the laboratory conducted the following experiment was performed**. 270 Kunming mice were divided into spleen group and spleen-free group. The spleen-free group was divided into the first spleen group and the spleen group, and then the spleen cells were inoculated and then transplanted into the spleen cell group. The spleen has an inhibitory effect on tumor growth in the early stage of tumor, and the inhibition rate is 25%. In the advanced stage of the tumor, the spleen progressively shrinks and loses its inhibitory effect. The spleen cell transplantation inhibits tumor growth, and its inhibition rate is 54%. The conclusion of this study is that the effect of spleen on tumor growth is biphasic, with some inhibition in the early stage and no inhibition in the late stage. Spleen cell transplantation can enhance the inhibition of tumor growth.

(2)   Experimental Study of exploring the impact of tumor on the thymus and spleen of the body's immune organs

The previous experimental studies have explored the effects of thymocytes of the central immune organs and peripheral immune organs on cancer cell transplantation and tumor growth. The findings and conclusions of the experimental results are as described above. Then, in turn, think about it further, what effect does the tumor have on the thymus and spleen of the immune organs? Therefore, the following experimental studies were carried out for further design. Forty Kunming mice were randomly divided into 4 groups, and the lymphocyte transformation rate was measured before the inoculation of cancer cells and on the 3rd, 7th and 14th day after inoculation of cancer cells. Thymus and spleen and other organs were observed and weighed and the slides of tissues were observed after execution.

It was found that in the early stage of tumor growth, the spleen was congested and swollen, and the cell proliferation was active. In the advanced stage of the tumor, the spleen showed progressive atrophy and cell proliferation was blocked. Immediately after inoculation of cancer cells, the thymus showed acute progressive atrophy, cell proliferation was blocked, the volume was significantly reduced, and the weight was significantly reduced, indicating that the cellular immune function was inhibited.

The results of this experiment suggest that the tumor will significantly inhibit the thymus, not only inhibiting thymus function, but also causing the immune organs to shrink.

(3)   Experimental Study of Exploring the anti-cancer effect of Chinese medicine Jianpi Yiqi Decoction

The above studies have found that the spleen has a certain influence on tumor growth, and spleen cell transplantation can increase the inhibition rate of tumors. Although the spleen referred to by Chinese medicine and the spleen referred to by Western medicine, these two are completely different in theory, pathogenesis and clinical. But this also reminds us that since they are all spleen, although they have different functions of the same name, can we use the law of spleen and qi, combined with the results of modern medical experiments, to form a compound of Chinese medicine for strengthening the spleen and replenishing qi, conducting animal experiments and observing whether or not it inhibits tumor function? 40 Kunming mice were divided into experimental group (n=30) and control group (n=10). The cells were inoculated with 0.1X 10^7 cells. The experimental group was continuously administered with Jianpi Yiqi Decoction for 14 days to observe the tumor growth, quality of life and survival of tumor-bearing mice.

The experimental results, taking Jianpi Yiqi Decoction can delay the emergence of tumor nodules after cancer cell transplantation, inhibit tumor growth, prolong the survival of tumor-bearing mice, and have a certain anti-cancer effect.

III, to explore the experimental study of the method of suppressing thymus atrophy and seeking immune reconstruction

In the manufacture of cancer-bearing animal models, the authors found that only thymectomy can be successfully modeled, and the same experiment was repeated in three batches. The results clearly demonstrated that the thymus has a definite relationship with tumorigenesis. In the above experimental study on the relationship between tumor and immune organs, the results clearly prove that the progression of the tumor can quickly make the thymus progressively atrophy, indicating that the tumor significantly inhibits the thymus, not only inhibits its function, but also causes the immune organ to shrink.

If this is the case, then we should use some methods to prevent the host's thymus from shrinking, restore the function of the thymus, and rebuild the immune system. Therefore, we further designed and wanted to use this immune device to transplant the immune cells to restore the immune organs, rebuild their organ function, and carry out experimental studies on the immune function of fetal liver, spleen and thymocytes transplanted. A group of 200 Kunming mice were used to make a subcutaneous solid tumor model of Hoai's ascites tumor. They were divided into 6 experimental groups and 2 control groups. The fetal spleen cells, fetal thymocytes and fetal liver cells were transplanted respectively. Tumor growth, regression, survival time, cellular immune index and histopathological examination were compared in mice. The results showed that the three groups of cells were transplanted together, the tumor regression rate was 40% in the near future, and the long-term tumor complete regression rate was 46.67%. The patients with complete tumor regression had long-term survival. The partial regression rate was 26.67% in the near term and 13.33% in the long term. The survival rate of some of the regressed people was extended by more than one month on average, the immune index was significantly improved, and the immune organs were hypertrophied. Tissue sections of the immune organs showed active cell growth. The results of this experiment show that the systemic adoptive immune reconstruction is partially reconstructed, and the overall system synergy can be used to better exert anti-tumor immune function and improve curative effect.

IV. Finding drugs that inhibit tumor angiogenesis from natural medicines

In 1986, when the author carried out cancer cell culture in the laboratory, it only promoted the proliferation of cancer cells, but it could not form a solid tumor mass. Later, it was discovered that if the chicken soup was dripped in the test tube cancer culture, it could promote the rapid growth of cancer cells. In a cluster, if 1 or 2 drops of aminophylline are dropped, it spreads quickly. **Since then, the author has been warning cancer patients not to eat chicken**. Currently, there are several steps in cancer cell metastasis. First, the cancer cells fall off, then invade the blood vessels into the blood, and the blood flow reaches the microcirculation and then releases the microvessels, reaches the metastatic organs, implants, first avascular stage, tumor Nodules, do not grow up, and soon form new blood vessels, tumors rapidly increase progress. In this transfer process, if one of the links can be blocked, the tumor metastasis can be prevented. The author considers the formation of neovascular microvessels in tumors, which is one of the key links in the transfer of cancer cells to rooting and growing into cancer nodules. Therefore, an experimental study on anti-tumor angiogenesis drugs from natural drugs was designed.

(I) Experimental study on the neovascularization of tumors in mice with abdominal muscle transplantation

Twenty Kunming mice were inoculated with EAC cell fluid in the abdominal muscles to prepare a new microvascular animal model of abdominal muscle transplantation. The Olympus microcirculation microscopy system was used to observe the neovascularization process and count the microvessel flow rate and flow rate. As a result, **it was found that there was no neovascularization on the first day after the inoculation, and on the second day, the neovascularization of the microvascular from the original host was observed to enter the tumor, and the neovascular density outside the tumor was increased in the third day.**

(II) Experimental study on the effects of different doses of Astragalus sinensis acetate extract (TG) on immune function in mice

Forty Kunming mice were randomly divided into TG1 group, TG2 group, TG3 group and TG4 group. The different doses of TG were administered for 12 days. On the 13th day, the rats in each group were sacrificed and the thymus and spleen were weighed. The results showed that different doses of TG had different effects on the immune organs of young rats. The thymus gland weight gain was observed at a small dose of 20 mg/kg, and the thymus gland was atrophied at a high dose of 80 mg/kg.

(III) Experimental study on the inhibitory effect of acetaminophen acetate extract (TG) on neovascularization of mouse abdominal muscle xenografts

40 Kunming mice were inoculated with EAC in the abdominal muscles to observe the neovascularization of abdominal muscle tumors. The mice were placed on the self-made observation platform, and the mouse observation table was placed on the microscope stage in the incubator. The morphology and number of neovascularization in the tumor and peritumoral were observed by HH-1 microcirculation detection system, and microscopic photographs were taken to measure the neovascular density of human tumors and the mean diameter and flow rate of the tumor.

The results showed that TG (20 mg/kg) significantly inhibited tumor angiogenesis in the early stage of tumors.

From the results of this group of experiments, it can be seen that TG can significantly inhibit the growth of neovascularization in the tumor and peritumoral, and reduce the density of new microvessels in human and tumor.

At present, scholars at home and abroad pay attention to try to inhibit tumor neovascularization to control tumor growth and metastasis formation. In May 1998, Folkman reported that his laboratory has developed two drugs that inhibit tumor neovascularization. For Angiostatin and Endostatin, in the tumor-bearing animal experiment, the tumor that transplanted the human body into the experimental mouse was significantly reduced. He used this anti-angiogenesis inhibitor to prevent blood vessel growth, atrophy of the capillary and cut off the nutritional supply of the tumor, thereby achieving treatment. The purpose of cancer. They reportedly planned to conduct very limited trials on the human body in 1999.

The author's laboratory completed the above-mentioned experimental study of TG in July 1997, because TG was originally a traditional Chinese medicine. This traditional Chinese medicine has been used in traditional Chinese medicine books for hundreds of years, and it has been applied in clinical practice for a long time. Not used to inhibit tumor neovascular growth. Therefore, since September 1998, the author has tried to use it as a comprehensive outpatient for anticancer and anti-metastasis treatment. It has been used in more than 80 patients with stage II and III cancer since December 1999. The preliminary observation of the efficacy of control, recurrence and metastasis is good and is currently in clinical validation observation.

3. Animal Discovery Research New Findings 2

Thymus atrophy and low immune function are one of the causes and pathogenesis of cancer

In order to explore the etiology, pathogenesis and pathophysiology of cancer, we conducted a series of animal experiments, from the results of experimental research to analyze and think, so that we can obtain new discoveries, new thinking, new enlightenment: one of the causes of cancer It may be atrophy of the thymus, impaired thymus function, and low immune function. Therefore, Professor XU ZE proposed one of the causes and pathogenesis of cancer at international conferences, which may be thymic atrophy, impaired central immune organ function, low immune function, decreased immune surveillance and immune escape. But what is the cause of the host's thymus atrophy? After repeated thoughts, it may be because a factor produced by solid tumors inhibits the thymus (Thymus), but this needs further study. We can temporarily call it "cancer Thymus inhibition factor or suppressor".

Looking back on the research history of cancer in the past 100 years, the research on the etiology, pathophysiology and pathogenesis of cancer is still rare. In the past 100 years, people have made efforts in clinical research and pathological research of cancer in the fields of surgery, radiotherapy and chemotherapy, but laboratory basic research and clinical basic research such as mutation, cloning, proliferation, metastasis, and planting regularity, such as invasion, metastasis, tumor thrombus, immunity, and endocrine, are relatively rare. Many large hospitals have not established laboratories for clinical basic research. Reviewing and reflecting on the experience and lessons of the author's clinical surgery for more than 60 years, it is clearly aware that if there was no breakthrough in clinical basic research, clinical efficacy is difficult to improve.

First, the new discovery of experimental research on the etiology, pathogenesis and pathophysiology of cancer

In the past 34 years, the author has carried out a series of experimental studies on animal experiments on the possible etiology, pathogenesis and pathophysiology of cancer, exploring the mechanisms of cancer invasion, recurrence and metastasis, and finding effective measures for regulation.

Experimental surgery is extremely important in the development of medical science. It is a key to opening the medical exclusion zone. Many disease prevention methods are applied to the clinic after many animal experiments have achieved stability results. Therefore, the author established an experimental surgical laboratory to conduct experimental tumor research, perform cancer cell transplantation, establish a tumor animal model, and carried out the following series of experimental tumor research:

1) Exploration of cancer etiology, pathogenesis, pathophysiology experimental research;
2) to explore cancer recurrence, metastasis mechanism and regularity;
3) to explore the relationship between tumor and immune and immune organs, and immune organs and tumors;
4) to explore the prevention of tumor progression, Methods for progressive atrophy and immune reconstitution of immune organs;
5) to find effective measures to regulate invasion, recurrence and metastasis of cancer.

Through experimental research and clinical practice experience, combined with the review, analysis, evaluation and self-reflection of traditional practice clinical practice cases over the past half century, the author summarizes the experience and lessons of the positive and negative aspects of clinical practice for more than 50 years. There are the following new discovery:

1. It was found from the results of follow-up

1) postoperative recurrence and metastasis are the key factors affecting the long-term efficacy of surgery. Clinicians must pay attention to and study the prevention and treatment of postoperative recurrence and metastasis in order to improve the long-term efficacy after

surgery. 2) Clinical basic research on recurrence and metastasis must be carried out. Without breakthroughs in basic research, clinical efficacy is difficult to improve.

2. It was found from the real tumor research

In order to explore the cause, pathogenesis, invasion and metastasis mechanism of cancer, and to find effective measures for regulation, intervention, recurrence and metastasis, the author and colleagues conducted a full four-year experimental tumor work.

(1) Experiment 1: Excision of mouse thymus (Thymus, TH) to produce a tumor-bearing animal model, injection of immunosuppressive drugs contribute to the establishment of a cancer-bearing animal model. The conclusions of the study prove that the occurrence and development of cancer have a significant correlation with the thymus and function of the host immune organs.

(2) Experiment 2: Whether it is immune first and then easy to get cancer, or cancer first and then low immunity, the experimental results confirmed that the first immune system is low and then easy to have cancer, the development, if no immune function decline, it is not easy to vaccinate success. The results suggest that improving and maintaining good immune function and protecting the central thymus gland is one of the important measures to prevent cancer.

(3) Experiment 3; In the study of the relationship between cancer metastasis and immunity, an animal model of liver metastasis cancer was established and divided into two groups, A and B. Group A used immunosuppressive drugs, and group B did not. Results The number of intrahepatic metastases in group A was significantly higher than that in group B. The experimental results suggest that metastasis is associated with immunity, low immune function or the use of immunosuppressive drugs to promote tumor metastasis.

(4) Experiment 4: When investigating the effect of tumor on immune organs, it was found that with the progress of cancer, the thymus showed progressive atrophy, and the host thymus was acute progressive atrophy after inoculation of cancer cells, and cell proliferation was blocked. The volume is significantly reduced. The results suggest that the tumor may inhibit the thymus and cause the immune organs to shrink.

(5) Experiment 5: It was found in the experiment that some of the experimental mice did not have a successful vaccination or the tumor grew very small, and the thymus did not significantly shrink. To understand the relationship between tumor and thymus atrophy, a group of experimental mice transplanted solid tumors were resected when they reached the size of the thumb. After 1 month of dissection, it was found that the thymus did not undergo progressive atrophy. Therefore, we speculate that it may be possible to develop a tumor that will not be known to inhibit the thymus, which needs further experimental research.

(6) Experiment 6: The above experimental results all prove that the progression of the tumor can cause progressive atrophy of the thymus, then can some methods be used to prevent

the host thymus from shrinking? Through animal experiments, we began to find ways or drugs to prevent thymocyte atrophy in tumor-bearing mice.

(6) Experiment 6:

The above experimental results have proved that the progression of the tumor can cause progressive atrophy of the thymus. So can some methods be used to prevent the host thymus from shrinking? Through animal experiments, we began to find ways or drugs to prevent thymus atrophy in tumor-bearing mice. The method of using the immune organ cell transplantation to restore the immune organ function was to inhibit tumor progression, immune organ atrophy and immune reconstruction. The experimental study on the immune function of fetal liver, fetal spleen and fetal thymocyte transplantation was performed by using mouse.

The results showed that the three groups of S, T, L cells were transplanted together, the tumor regression rate was 40% in the near future, and the long-term tumor complete regression rate was 46.67%. The tumor completely disappeared and survived for a long time.

(7) Experiment 7: In the experiment of investigating the effect of tumor on the spleen of the immune organs of the body, it was found that the spleen had an inhibitory effect on tumor growth in the early stage of the tumor, and in the late stage of the tumor, the spleen also showed progressive atrophy. The results suggest that the effect of spleen on tumor growth is bi-directional, with some inhibition in the early stage and no inhibition in the late stage. Spleen cell transplantation can enhance the inhibition of tumors.

(8) Experiment 8: Follow-up results suggest that controlled metastasis is the key to cancer treatment. It is currently known that there are many steps and links in cancer cell metastasis. In order to block one of the links to prevent its metastasis, it is believed that tumor neovascularization may be one of the links in which cancer cells can be implanted into a cancerous nodule. In 1986, the author carried out the research work of microcirculation, and observed the microvessel formation and flow velocity of transplanted tumor nodules in mice bearing mice with microcirculation microscope, and then searched for anti-tumor angiogenesis drugs from natural drugs. The Olympus microcirculation microscopy system was used to observe the process of neovascularization and count the flow rate of micro-arteries and venules, and to extract the TG from the genus. As a result, no neovascularization was observed on the first day of inoculation, and microscopic neovascularization was observed on the second day. TG can reduce the density of new microvessels in human tumors.

(9) Experiment 9: Some of the solid tumors inoculated subcutaneously from a large number of tumor-bearing animal models in the laboratory grew larger, and the cancer cells of the central tissue structure were different from the surrounding cancer cells. Most of the centers are sterile necrosis or liquefaction, and the surrounding areas are still active cancer cells. Therefore, in the clinical treatment work, the treatment of sterile necrosis can be taken.

Second, to explore ways to curb tumor progression, progressive atrophy of thymus and immune reconstruction

The above experimental studies suggest that one of the causes of cancer and the pathogenesis may be thymus atrophy, thymocyte proliferation is blocked, thymus function is impaired, immune function is low, and the immune escape of malignant cells is caused.

Since the thymus will undergo a progressive atrophy as the tumor progresses, how can it be done to prevent it from shrinking? Animal experiments were conducted to find ways or drugs to prevent thymic atrophy in tumor-bearing mice. Eventually, immune organ cell transplantation was used to restore the function of the immune organ, and exciting results were obtained.

At that time, the author had considered the above experimental methods for clinical trials, attempting to use the water cells to induce the thymus homogenate to test the same kind of thymocyte transplantation, but medical ethics is not allowed, so it was not implemented.

In 1986, at the satellite conference of the International Microcirculation Conference, the author was inspired to find ways to improve microcirculation drugs from natural medicines.

From biological cell transplantation, adoptive immunization reconstitutes the immune system, and then seeks to activate cytokines from natural medicines such as Chinese herbal medicines, enhance immune surveillance, thereby inhibiting tumors and preventing thymus atrophy. All drugs must pass animal experiments and clinical validation, so after 3 years in the study of cancer-bearing animal models, 20 will be from natural drugs. A variety of traditional Chinese medicines were used to conduct anti-cancer immune control Chinese medicines. It was screened by clinical observation and verified, and further filtered and concentrated into $XZ-C_{1-10}$ from traditional Chinese medicine immunopharmacology, or anti-cancer immune regulation and control chinese medicine, which can promote thymic hyperplasia, prevent thymus atrophy, enhance immune function, protect bone marrow, promote T lymphocyte function and cytokines, and have a high tumor inhibition rate, only inhibit cancer cells. Does not affect normal cells and can be taken orally for a long time. Because cancer is a chronic disease, the division, proliferation, and cloning of cancer cells are long-term, continuous, and progressive. Therefore, it is advisable to use a sustained-release drug that can be used for a long time, is non-toxic, and can be taken orally. Chinese herbal medicine treatment of cancer is to treat the cause and pathogenesis from the overall perspective of human beings. It not only kills cancer cells, but also enhances the body›s autoimmune function, thereby enhancing the body›s anti-cancer ability, so it can make some refractory and extensive. The metastasis of cancer can be controlled, prolonging the lives of cancer patients, alleviating the suffering of patients, and opening up a path worthy of further exploration for cancer treatment.

On December 12, 2009, the author was invited to an academic exchange visit to the Sterling Cancer Institute in Hughes, USA.

Founded in 1969, the Institute is an 86-year-old professor. One of the company's main research results was the earliest international invention of Swiss hairless immune mice for cancer research and become the standard animal model for cancer research in the United States. In the early 1970s, scientists first implanted human tumors into athymic mice and made major research breakthroughs. Dr. Giov-anella of the institute also participated. Studies have shown that athymic mice are ideal experimental animals with weak immune system and no resistance to tumors. In the early 1970s, scientists first implanted human tumors into athymic mice and made major research breakthroughs. Dr. Giov-anella of the institute also participated. **Studies have shown that athymic mice are ideal experimental animals with weak immune systems and no resistance to tumors.**

From the Stirling Cancer Institute, athymic nude mice have been found to be animal models of transplanted cancer. In recent years, animal experiments in various countries have so far determined that **athymic nude mice have been the gold standard for studying cancer treatment animal models**.

The results of a series of animal experiments on the etiology, pathogenesis and pathophysiology of cancer suggest that thymectomy leads to immunodeficiency, and then immune surveillance declines, eventually developing into immune escape, which may be one of the key causes of pain and pathogenesis. It is a new development of 21st century oncology theory, which provides direction and basis for cancer therapeutics in the 21st century, and provides theoretical basis and experimental basis for cancer immune regulation and targeted therapy. This innovation has not been mentioned in textbooks and literature at home and abroad.

Once the above theory and doctrine have been demonstrated and recognized, it will lead to a series of changes and updates in cancer therapeutics, such as changes and updates in the understanding of the concept of cancer treatment, changes and updates in the understanding of cancer treatment goals or targets, and diagnosis of cancer, changes and updates in methodological and therapeutic criteria, changes and updates in cancer treatment methods and treatment models; changes and updates in the research and development of anticancer and anti-metastatic drugs.

4. Animal Discovery Research New Findings 3

The theoretical basis and experimental basis of xz-c immune regulation and control therapy with "protection of Thymus and Increase of Immune function"

I, the animal experiment enlightenment

The researchers in the laboratory of the author found that the thymus of the cancer-bearing mice showed progressive atrophy, and the central immune organs were damaged, and should be protected by "protecting Thymus and increasing Immune."

Based on the implications of experimental research on the etiology and pathogenesis of cancer, Professor Xu Ze first proposed a new theory and method for XZ-C immunomodulation targeted therapy. As a result of experimental research, it was found that the thymus of the cancer-bearing mice showed progressive atrophy, and the central immune organ function was impaired, the immune function was decreased, and the immune surveillance was low.

Therefore, the treatment principle must be to prevent progressive atrophy of the thymus and promote thymic hyperplasia, and to protect bone marrow hematopoietic function, to have improve immune surveillance, and to control immune escape of malignant cells.

It is well known that immune organs have central immune organs and peripheral immune organs. The former includes the thymus and bone marrow, and the latter includes the spleen and lymph nodes. It has been confirmed that when a cancer occurs, a factor that suppresses the immune organs (**we temporarily call it a cancer suppressor (free) factor**) inhibits the thymus, causes the thymus to gradually shrink, the central immune function is inhibited, and the immune function is reduced. To make the immune surveillance weakened or missing, the tumor will inevitably develop further.

After more than 34 years of clinical trials and observations of more than 12,000 patients with advanced cancer in 34 years of oncology clinics, the author has confirmed that the treatment principle of Thymus protection and Increase Immune function enhancement is correct and reasonable, and the curative effect is satisfactory.

XZ-C (Xu ZE-China) immunomodulatory therapy was first proposed by Professor Xu Ze in China in 2006 in his book "New Concepts and New Methods for Cancer Metastasis Treatment". He believes that under normal circumstances, there is a dynamic balance between cancer and body defense. The occurrence and development of cancer is caused by the imbalance of dynamic balance. If the condition that has been dysregulated is adjusted to a normal level, the growth of the cancer can be controlled and allowed to subside.

It is well known that the occurrence and development of cancer and its prognosis are determined by the comparison of two factors, namely, the biological characteristics of cancer cells and the host body's own ability to control cancer cells. If the two are balanced, the tumor can be controlled, and if the two are out of balance, the cancer develops.

Under normal circumstances, the host's body itself has certain restrictions on cancer cells, but in the case of cancer, these restrictive defenses will be inhibited and damaged to varying degrees, resulting in cancer cells losing immune surveillance and cancer cell immunity. However, in the case of cancer, these restraining abilities will be inhibited and damaged to varying degrees. Thereby causing the cancer cells to lose their immune surveillance, and cancer cell immune escape occurs, and the cancer cells are further developed and metastasized.

II, it should protect, regulate and activate the anticancer immune system in the human body.

When discussing the principles of cancer treatment, we should study what anti-cancer immune cell series are in the human body, what anti-cancer cell factor series are, what anti-cancer gene series are, and which humoral immunity series are.

1. What anti-cancer immune cells in the human body may be activated and enhanced to prevent cancer cell metastasis

(1)   Cytotoxic lymphocytes (CTL):

It plays a major role in anti-tumor immunity. Human CTL cells are CD3 and CD8. CTL cells are high in peripheral blood and spleen, and also have a certain content in thoracic duct, thymus and bone marrow. Under certain conditions, IL-2, 1L-4, IFN and other cytokines can also be produced, and other anti-cancer immune cells, killing macrophages, natural killer cells and killer B cells can be activated to exert anti-tumor effects.

(2)   Natural killer cells (NK cells):

NK cells are a group of broad-spectrum anti-cancer cells whose killing activity is independent of antibodies and does not depend on the thymus. Its main function is to monitor and eliminate cancerous cells in the human body. Clinical observations have shown that the incidence of malignant tumors is significantly increased in people with defective NK cell activity, and NK cells are an important part of the early anti-cancer immune surveillance function of the body.

(3)   LAK cells:

LAK cells are the most important anti-cancer cells in modern biological therapy. Human peripheral monocytes (PBMNC) can significantly kill a variety of tumor cells in vitro induced by IL-2 in vitro. LAK cells have a broader spectrum of tumor killing than NK cells and can also kill tumor cells that NK cells cannot kill.

(4)   Macrophages (M. cells):

It plays an important role in the body's anti-tumor immunity.
2. What anti-disease cytokines are activated and enhanced in the human body for cancer metastasis

(1)   Interferon (IFN):

Interferon is resistant to cell differentiation and has immunomodulatory functions. It has anti-proliferative effects on certain tumor cells, and its anti-cancer effect may be related to immune regulation. It can make NK cells and M. Increased cell viability.

(2)   Interleukin-2 (IL-2):

It is a T cell growth factor with strong immunoregulatory function, which promotes the activation of T cells, NK cells and monocytes, and also promotes the release of IFN-a and TNF.

(3)   Tumor necrosis factor (TNF):

Its effect on cells is cytotoxic and can affect the microvessels of the tumor, eventually leading to necrosis at the center of the tumor.

3. other

In recent years, due to the rapid development of molecular biology, molecular immunology, molecular immunopharmacology, and genetic engineering, the basic and clinical research of the molecular level of "anti-cancer institutions" has been expanding and deepening. The research prospects of anti-cancer and anti-metastasis are very gratifying.

At present, research on anti-cancer molecular biological immunotherapy mainly focuses on four subsystems of anti-cancer institutions, namely anti-cancer therapy, anti-cancer factor therapy, anti-cancer gene therapy and anti-cancer antibody therapy.

The basic feature of these molecular biology and molecular immunotherapy is that all preparations of molecular biological immunotherapy are the **organism's own substances**, which differ from the roots of radiotherapy and chemotherapy in that it is normal to the body's normal tissue cells, especially The cells and functions of the immune system and the structure and function of the bone marrow hematopoietic system not only have no progressive damage, but also have immune response regulation and enhancement. It is well known that radiotherapy and chemotherapy are non-selective "injury therapy". Killing cancer cells also kills normal cells, which damages normal tissues of the body and damages the structure and function of the bone marrow hematopoietic system and immune system, leading to serious consequences.

Biological therapy is a therapy that stabilizes and balances the life mechanism through regulation of biological responses. American scholar Oldham proposed the theory of biological regulation in 1984, and then proposed the concept of tumor biological therapy.

III. Overview of research on biology regulator-like anti-cancer traditional Chinese medicines

XZ-C immunomodulation anti-cancer Chinese medicine has been confirmed by animal experiments and clinical practice to have biological modulator-like effects and curative effects, and is a drug selected from natural medicine resources.

The experimental screening work was mainly carried out by the in vivo anti-tumor experiment of the tumor-bearing animal model. One experimental group of traditional Chinese medicine was observed. The animal model was observed for 3 months, and 48 effective anti-cancer Chinese herbal medicines were selected for each 2 or 3 flavors. In vivo anti-tumor experiments of tumor-bearing animals were carried out. It was found that the anti-tumor experiment of single-flavor Chinese medicine was not as good as the anti-tumor effect of the compound anti-tumor experiment of multi-flavored traditional Chinese medicine, and the single-flavor Chinese medicine only inhibited the proliferation of tumors. The compound combination of multi-flavored traditional Chinese medicine not only inhibits the tumor growth of tumor-bearing animals, but also has a good regulation effect on immune regulation, enhancement of physical strength, enhancement of immune function, promotion of tumor cell cytokine production and protection of normal cells.

In the in vitro experimental screening of 4 years of single-flavored traditional Chinese medicine and the screening of tumor-bearing animal models in vivo, the experimental combination was optimized, and then the experiment was reconstituted to XZ-C1-10 immunomodulation anti-cancer, anti-metastatic, anti-relapse combination, and finally clinical validation.

Since 1992, the author has organized a collaborative group to carry out clinical verification. After more than 30 years of clinical verification and observation of more than 12,000 patients with various cancers in the Dawn Cancer Specialized Clinic, the patients have stable, improved symptoms, improved symptoms and improved quality of life. The survival period is significantly extended. Many patients who have metastasized stabilized the lesion after administration, and the cancer cells did not spread or metastasize further. Some patients could not undergo radiotherapy or chemotherapy for reasons such as decreased white blood cell count after surgery, and the metastasis was controlled after taking the drug, and no metastasis was performed.

IV. Biological response modifier-like action and efficacy Of XZ-C traditional Chinese medicine immunomodulation

The regulation of biological responses was first described by Oldham in 1982. The implication is the ability to regulate the body's response or response to external "attacks" through biological response modifiers (BRMs).

The cytokines and humoral factors of the body's immune system are in a delicate regulation. In the case of imbalance, the body's response or response ability will be significantly affected. The use of biological response modifiers is to restore the unbalanced body state to a normal equilibrium state for the purpose of disease prevention.

BRM opens up new areas of cancer biotherapy. At present, BRM is widely regarded as the fourth mode of cancer treatment by the medical community.

The biological response modifier has the function of regulating the immune function of the body and restoring the suppressed immune system of the body. The mechanism of action is multifaceted, but no matter what mechanism, it plays its regulatory function by activating the body's immune system.

Biological response modifiers, often referred to as microbial and plant sources, have previously been referred to as immunopotentiators, immune cordials, immunostimulants or immunomodulators and are now collectively designated as biological response modifiers or modifiers.

In the laboratory, the xz-c immunoregulatory anti-cancer anti-metastatic Chinese medicine, which has been successfully screened by tumor-bearing mice in the laboratory, has improved immunity, protects the central immune system thymus, enhances cellular immunity, and protects thymus tissue function. Improve immunity, protect bone marrow blood production, increase red blood cell and white blood cell count, activate immune cytokines, and improve immune surveillance in the blood. The main pharmacological action of xz-c immunomodulation anticancer Chinese medicine is to protect Thymus and to increase Immune function. After 48 years of animal experiments, 48 kinds of single traditional Chinese medicines with higher tumor inhibition rate were detected by immunological and cytokine levels. 26 of them had enhanced phagocytosis, enhanced cellular immunity, or enhanced humoral immunity, or increase the weight of the thymus, or promote the proliferation of bone marrow cells, or enhance the function of T cells, or enhance the activity of LAK cells, or inhibit platelet coagulation and antithrombotic, or anti-tumor, anti-metastasis, or scavenge free radicals. Summarize the mechanism of xz-c immune regulation and control of anticancer Chinese medicine as follows.

1. Activate the body's immune cell system, promote the enhancement of the host defense mechanism, and restore the ability to respond to cancer.
2. Activate the immune cytokine system of the body's anti-cancer mechanism, enhance the host's immune defense mechanism, and improve the immune surveillance of immune cells in the body's blood circulation system.
3. Protect the thymus, enhance immunity, protect the marrow from blood, protect the physiological mechanism of the epiphysis, stimulate the bone marrow hematopoietic function, promote the recovery of bone marrow function, and increase the white blood cell and red blood cell count.
4. Reduce the adverse reactions of radiotherapy and chemotherapy, and enhance the tolerance of the host.
5. The progression of cancer is caused by the imbalance between the biological characteristics of cancer cells and the body's ability to inhibit cancer. The role of xz-c immunoregulation is to improve immunity and restore balance.
6. It can directly regulate the growth and differentiation of tumor cells, and regulate the growth and differentiation.
7. Can increase the thymus, increase weight, and make the thymus no longer atrophy.
8. Stimulate the host's anti-tumor immune response, enhance the body's anti-tumor ability, enhance the sensitivity of cancer cells to the body's anti-cancer mechanism, and help to kill cancer cells in the process of metastasis.

XZ-C immunomodulation Chinese medicine treatment of tumors can enable the host to produce a strong immune response to cancer cells, thereby achieving the purpose of treating cancer. XZ-C immunomodulation anticancer Chinese medicine can cause the following immunological reactions in the host: 1 enhance the regulation or restore the host's immune response to the tumor; 2 stimulate the body's inherent immune function, activate the host's immune defense system; 3 restore immune function.

As mentioned above, the mechanism of action of XZ-C immunomodulation anticancer Chinese medicine is similar to BRM, and the clinical use also has the same therapeutic effect as BRM.

5. Clinical application principles and scope of application of xz-c immunomodulatory Chinese medicine

(1) Principles of application of XZ-C immunomodulatory Chinese medicine

BRM and BRM-like XZ-C immunomodulation anticancer Chinese medicine can enhance the body's immune response and strengthen the body's tumor immune surveillance. When the cells are mutated or the tumor is small, the effect is better. The best results are achieved when the tumor is reduced to a minimum by surgery or radiation therapy or medication. For those who have lost the chance of surgery, poor physical fitness, can not tolerate radiotherapy, chemotherapy, immunotherapy has a certain effect, can alleviate symptoms and prolong the survival time of patients. After radical resection of the tumor, in order to reduce recurrence and metastasis, it is feasible to treat xz-c with traditional Chinese medicine. After surgical resection of large tumors, XZ-C is also feasible to eliminate cancer cells that may remain and distant cancer cells. Immune regulation of traditional Chinese medicine treatment. If the tumor can not be removed, radiotherapy or chemotherapy can be performed first, and the tumor cells are most killed, so that the tumor burden in the body is reduced, and then XZ-C immunomodulation is used to treat the Chinese medicine.

(2) Clinical observation and application range of xz-c immunomodulatory Chinese medicine

1. Post-cancer metastasis. Restore and improve postoperative immunity, improve postoperative survival quality, kill residual cancer cells, inhibit cancer cell proliferation, prevent metastasis, recurrence, consolidate and enhance long-term efficacy.

Scope of application: 1 after all kinds of advanced radical cancer surgery; 2 after palliative resection of various cancers; 3 exploration can not be removed after advanced cancer surgery; 4 can only do gastrointestinal anastomosis or colostomy; 5 late The cancer has been unable to be removed, and the surgical indication is lost; 6 tumor resection + intubation pump.

2. Comprehensively improve the quality of life of patients with advanced cancer, prolong survival, inhibit cancer cell mitosis, control cancer cell proliferation, improve overall immunity, and resist proliferation and metastasis.

Scope of application: 1 recent or long-term metastasis after various cancer surgery, or recurrence; 2 liver metastases of various advanced cancers, lung metastasis, brain metastasis, or with cancerous pleural effusion, cancerous ascites.

3. Relieve cancer pain. Oral or external application of xz-c Chinese medicine can treat the advanced cancer intractable pain, and soften and reduce the body surface metastatic mass.

4. It can protect the immune organs such as liver, kidney, bone marrow hematopoietic system and thymus with the treatment of infusion or intubation pump, improve immunity, improve the overall immune status after drug treatment, maintain, consolidate and enhance the efficacy of intermittent and long-term medication. To prevent metastasis, spread, recurrence, comprehensively improve and improve the quality of life after liver cancer patients and other interventions or intubation treatment, and prolong survival.

5. Combined with radiotherapy and chemotherapy, it can alleviate adverse reactions, enhance treatment effects, protect liver, kidney, bone marrow hematopoietic system and immune organs, improve immune function, and increase white blood cell count.

6. XZC immunomodulation anticancer traditional Chinese medicine combined with traditional Chinese medicine decoction, such as combined with anti-cancer Shugan Xiaoshui Decoction, treating liver cancer with ascites or abdominal metastatic cancerous ascites; combined with Huihuang Decoction, treating liver cancer with jaundice; In combination with Jiangai Decoction, the treatment of liver cancer with high transaminase and HBsAg-positive patients; combined with Shengxue Decoction, treatment of chemotherapy-induced leukopenia.

(3) The timing of application of XZ-C immunomodulation anticancer Chinese medicine

Cancer patients are mostly immunocompromised, and should be treated immediately after diagnosis. The three major treatments of surgery, radiotherapy and chemotherapy may promote the patient's immune function, which will reduce the patient's endurance to surgery or chemotherapy and radiotherapy. And reduce the immune surveillance function in the immune cell system of the patient's body. Therefore, immunotherapy should be performed during the operation or at the beginning of the radiotherapy or chemotherapy period.

XZ-C immunomodulatory chinese medicine is an oral drug, as long as the patient can eat orally can take oral XZ-C Chinese medicine. Continued administration of XZ-C immunomodulatory Chinese medicine for a period of time after radiotherapy, chemotherapy, radiotherapy, chemotherapy, and radiotherapy and chemotherapy can help reduce or control recurrence and metastasis, reduce adverse reactions of radiotherapy and chemotherapy, and prevent chemotherapy. It leads to low immune function and enhances immunity, promotes bone marrow blood production, protects the marrow from blood, activates the body's immune cell system and immune cytokine system, improves immune surveillance, and prevents recurrence and metastasis.

5. Animal Discovery Research New Findings 4

Experimental observation on the effect of tumor on thymus and spleen of immune organs

It is generally believed that the immune function of the body affects the occurrence, development and prognosis of the tumor, and the tumor also has an inhibitory effect on the immune state of the body. Both are the mutual cause and effect and it is complex. In the animal experiment of the effect of spleen on tumor growth, it was observed that many changes occurred in the thymus and spleen of the immune organs of tumor-bearing mice. It seems that there is a certain rule in the meantime. In order to further explore the relationship between tumor and spleen and thymus and its regularity, the following experiment was designed to dynamically observe the changes of thymus, spleen and lymphocyte transformation rate of tumor-bearing mice in different periods for exploring the regularity between them.

[Materials and Methods】

1. Experimental animals and grouping

Forty Kunming mice were randomly divided into 4 groups. The mice were 40-50 days old and weighed 15-18 g.

Group I: healthy control group, healthy mice that were not inoculated with cancer cells, and the thymus, spleen and peripheral blood were taken for observation after sacrifice.

Group II: Inoculation of Ehrlich ascites tumor cells by intraperitoneal cavity was 0.1 XIO7, and sacrificed after 3 days.

Group Ill: Inoculated with cancer cells (ibid.), and observed on the 7th day.

Group IV: On the 14th day of inoculation of cancer cells, observation was performed.

Take the experiment in the previous data (the experimental study on the effect of spleen on tumor growth). The results of autopsy after 100 natural deaths in tumor-bearing mice, as a result of changes in thymus and spleen of advanced tumor, thymus in late stage tumor-bearing mice The average diameter is (1.2 ± 0.3) mm, the average weight is (20 ± 5) mg, and the texture is hard. However, the spleen is extremely atrophied, and the average weight is (60 ± 12) mg. The texture is hard, the color is gray, the germinal center is significantly reduced, and fibrosis occurs.

2, experimental methods

Each group of mice was sacrificed by excretion of the eyeball at the scheduled time. Each mouse was given whole blood (heparin anticoagulation) irnl for lymphocyte transformation test, and then the mice were immediately dissected to observe the tumor infiltration range and ascites volume. And the involvement of various organs, and focus on the anatomy of the thymus, spleen and lymph nodes, and completely remove the thymus and spleen, measure the volume with a vernier caliper, and then send the disease by weighing the analytical balance.

3. Determination of peripheral blood lymphocyte transformation rate in each group of mice

It was determined by micro blood volume whole blood morphology method. Dig the eyeball to take the whole blood, heparin anticoagulation.

4. Tumor model preparation is the same as the experimental part in the previous data

[Experimental results]

1. The weight of the thymus in different periods after the mice were inoculated with cancer cells is shown in Table 1.

The variance analysis was performed on Table 1, see Table 2. The results of Tables 1 and 2 are shown by curves, and the thymus weight change curve (Fig. 1) is plotted. The weight of the thymus on the 25th and 30th days in the figure is derived from the experimental results in the previous.

Table 1 Comparison of thymic weights of mice in each group (mg)

Group	Group I healthy	Group II on the 3rd after inoculated	Group III on the 7th after inoculated	Group IV on the 14th after inoculated

组别	I 组正常组	II 组接种后第 3 天	III 组接种后第 7 天	N 组接种后第 14 天		
	72.8	78.2	90.0	40.0		
	50.0	83.4	66.0	32.2		
	56.4	89	85.4	39.8		
	96.4	68	106.5	23.5		
	77.4	74.8	51.7	38.0		
X_i	100.7	95.4	77.8	36.0		
	87.5	115.0	73.0	16.0		
	76.8	56.4	60.0	20.0		
	112.7	43.0	49.4	55		
	51.0			20		
$\sum X$	781.07	703.2	736.3	350.5	$\sum X$	2 571.7
N_i	10	9	10	10	N	39
$\bar{X_i}$	78.17	78.13	73.63	35.05	$\bar{X}$	65.94
$\sum_i X_i^2$	6 6261.79	58 566.66	57 033.75	18 467.25	$\sum X^2$	191 324.75

Table 2 analyzes the variance of Table 1

Resources of variation	SS	V	MS	F	P
Between groups	12967.10	3	4322.36	12.85	<0.01
Within groups	11777.12	35	336.48		
Total	24744.22	38			

As can be seen from Table 1, Table 2, and Figure 1, the thymus of the tumor-bearing mice showed a regular change. Within 7 days after inoculation, there was no significant change in the thymus macroscopic view, but the weight had begun to decrease. After the large, there is an acute progressive atrophy. The diameter of each leaf of the late thymus is reduced from the normal 5--8mm to about 1mm, and the weight is reduced from 76.1mg to 20mg. The texture becomes hard and the function is also reduced or even lost. It indicates that the cellular immune function of the body is increasingly manipulated and inhibited as the tumor progresses, causing the immune function to be low, and the tumor growth is getting faster and faster.

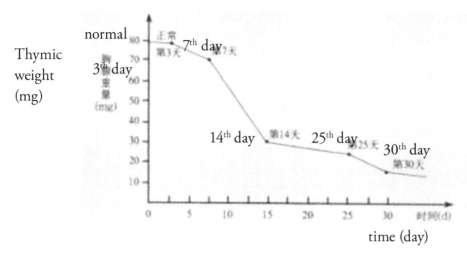

Fig1. the curve of variation on the thymic weights

2. The changes of spleen weight in each group of tumor-bearing mice at different times are shown in Table 3 and Table 4.

Table 3 splenic weights of cancer-bearing mice in each group in different phases

Group	Group I healthy	Group II on the 3rd after inoculated	Group III on the 7th after inoculated	Group IV on the 14th after inoculated

组别	I 组正常组	II 组接种后第 3 天	III 组第 7 天		IV 组第 14 天
	98.4	103.0	152.8		120.7
	86.0	110.3	175.8		96.9
	139.0	153.2	154.5		103.0
	126.0	96.7	154.0		102.0
	194.4	206.0	290.4		91.0
X_i	130	137.0	156.9		122.3
	107.4	174.0	184.0		88.6
	82.8	143.0	232.0		109.0
	86.0	160	86.3		192.4
	82.0				119.0
ΣX	1 258.4	1 205.0	1 720.9	1 021 ΣX	5 210.2
N_i	10	9	9	10 N	38
$\bar{X}$	125.84	134.43	172.09	102.1 $\bar{X}$	133.59
ΣX^2	169 020.88	175 088.97	322 834.65	106.41 ΣX^2	773.385

Resources of variation	SS	V	MS	F	P
Between groups	25345.12	3	8448	5.68	<0.01
Within groups	51983	35	1485.24		
Total	77328.12	38			

Table 4 Analysis of variance of table 23-3

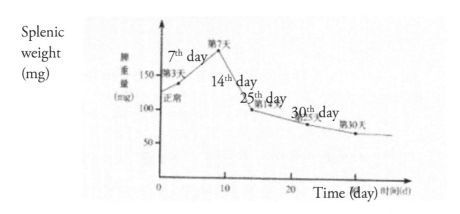

Fig. 2 the curve of variation on the splenic weights

For the autopsy of 100 mice in the experimental group in the previous data, the average weight of the spleen was 60 ± 12 mg, and the spleen heavy star was changed to make a curve description.

From Table 3 and Table 4. Figure 2, it can be seen that the spleen of tumor-bearing mice gradually increases in size and gains weight in the early stage.

In the later stage, it is progressively atrophied. It is indicated that in the early stage of tumor, due to tumor stimulation, cell proliferation is active, the immune response effect is enhanced, and the anti-tumor effect is also enhanced, thereby exerting a role in inhibiting tumor growth. In the late stage, due to the large increase in the number of tumors, a large number of inhibitory cells and immunosuppressive factors are produced, which hinders the proliferation of spleen immune cells, consumes effector cells, and causes atrophy, fibrous tissue proliferation, inhibition or disappearance of tumor suppressing effects, and even promotes tumor growth.

3. Comparison of peripheral blood lymphocyte transformation test results in tumor-bearing mice at different times See Table 5, Table 6

Table 5 Comparison of lymphocyte transformation rate of lymphocyte transformation test in each group at different times (%)

Group I healthy	Group II on the 3rd after inoculated	Group III on the 7th after inoculated	Group IV on the 14th after inoculated

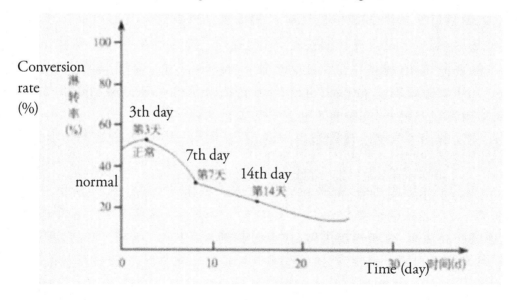

	组正常组		组接种后第3天		组第7天		组第14天
	45		53		43		31
	40		62		32		28
	51		48		26		19
	42		43		45		21
	60		52		30		22
	39		51		32		23
			50				
ΣX	277	359	208	144	ΣX		988
N_i	6	7	6	6	N		25
$\bar{X_i}$	46,17	51,29	24		$\bar{X}$		39,52
$\Sigma_i X$	13 111	18 611	7 498	3 560	ΣX^2		42 780

Table 6 Analysis of variance of table 5

Using a curve to present the results of table5 and table 6, draw the curve of lymphocyte conversion rate of the cancer-bearing mice at different time (Fig. 3).

Figure 3 The curve of Lymphocyte conversion rate

As can be seen from Table 5, Table 6 and Figure 3, the lymphocyte transformation rate of the pain-bearing mice also showed a certain regularity, which increased slightly after inoculation, followed by an acute progressive decline to the post-inoculation. In 14th days (late), the conversion rate dropped to about 50% of normal, and continued to decline in the future, indicating that the tumor has an inhibitory effect on the cellular immunity of the machine during the whole course of disease, and the inhibition occurs as the disease progresses. The stronger the effect, the more immune function is damaged.

From Fig.1, 2 and 3 it can be known that the changes in thymic volume and weight are extremely similar to the curve of lymphocyte conversion rate presented as synchronism. By contrast, the changes in splenic volume and weight are different from them with increase in the early period and the decrease, which indicates that during the middle and later period, both the organismal humoral immunity and cellular immunity are damaged and inhibited.

4. Pathological changes of thymus and spleen

(1)thymus:

showing progressive atrophy throughout the course of the disease, on the third day after inoculation of cancer cells, the thymus is slightly reduced, the color is slightly gray, on the 7th day after inoculation, the thymus volume is earlier Significantly atrophy, cell proliferation is blocked, mature cells are reduced, and to the advanced stage of the tumor, the thymus is extremely atrophied, the volume is about the size of sesame seeds, the diameter is 1mm, and the texture becomes hard.

(2) Spleen:

In the early stage of the tumor, the congestion is swollen and the volume is increased. Large, dark red, crisp, increased germinal center, and fewer mature cells. On the 14th day after inoculation, the spleen also showed progressive atrophy, reduced volume, grayish gray, hard, reduced germinal center, and blocked cell proliferation. There are few mature cells and fibrosis develops until fibrosis.

[Discuss]

1. The effect of tumor on the structure and function of spleen

The results of this experiment show that the tumor affects the immune function of the body, and the spleen of the tumor-bearing mice will change regularly. In the early stage of spleen hyperplasia, cell proliferation is active, germinal center is increased, mature cells are increased, and the effect of inhibiting tumor growth is exerted. The advanced spleen is progressively atrophied, cell proliferation is limited, germinal center is reduced, and fibrotic tissue is fibrotic. The texture hardens and loses its anti-tumor immunity. The spleen has such a change, and its mechanism is still unclear. It needs to be further explored. It may be speculated that on the one hand, tumor cells stimulate the host immune system through tumor-specific antigens, and stimulate immune effects to kill tumor cells and protect the body. On the other hand, tumor cells can induce inhibition

Immune cells (mainly T-suppressor cells and macrophages) and the production of inhibitory factors, together with the tumor cells themselves secrete many immunosuppressive factors, thereby inhibiting the body's immune anti-cancer effect, escaping the immune killing monitoring effect and survival and development, the spleen is The body's largest peripheral lymphoid organs, the body fluid molecule Tuftisin, which produces immune lymphocytes and antibodies, and produces anti-tumor effects. When cancer cells invade the body early, the spleen is stimulated to react, the cells proliferate actively, and the function is strong, producing more immune effect cells and lymphokines to inhibit tumor growth. In the late stage, due to the progression of the tumor, a large number of immunosuppressive factors are produced, resulting in spleen atrophy, limited function or damage, thereby losing the positive effect of anti-tumor immunity.

2. About the impact of tumors on the thymus

The experimental results showed that after inoculation of cancer cells, the thymus was immediately suppressed, and the whole process was progressively atrophied, so the thymus quickly lost the anti-tumor immune effect. It was observed in the experiment that the thymus gland undergoes a change in morphological structure shortly after inoculation of the cancer cells, and the entire course of the disease is progressively atrophied. By the end of the tumor, the weight of the thymus was reduced from 78.13 ± 13.2 mg to 20 ± 5 mg, and the volume was reduced from a diameter of 5-'Smm to 1 mm. Cell proliferation was significantly blocked.

Due to progressive atrophy of the thymus, cell proliferation is blocked, mature cells are reduced or depleted, the index is decreased, metabolism is weakened, cell viability is decreased, and thymus hormone secretion is also reduced. The cellular immune function of the body is inevitably damaged, and the defense ability of the mouse is low. The transplanted human cancer cells grow and multiply. Zhang Tongwen and other similar reports have found that the thymus atrophy of tumor-bearing mice is accompanied by the inhibition of bone ft cell proliferation and the decrease of nucleated cell viability, and it is considered that there is a close relationship between the two. It can be seen that the inhibition or damage effect of the tumor on the host immune function is multifaceted, affecting the entire immune system of the body. The lymphocyte transformation rate test of this group showed that the lymphocyte transformation rate decreased progressively after inoculation of cancer cells, and decreased to more than 50% in the late stage, indicating that the cellular immune effect was inhibited. As for why the thymus of tumor-bearing mice is inhibited and atrophied, further experimental research and observation are needed. In order to achieve immune function, vertebrates have evolved to have a special lymphatic network distributed throughout the body, and the entire immune system consists of central lymphoid organs and peripheral lymphoid organs. The thymus is an important central lymphoid organ that promotes T cell differentiation and maturation to exert cellular immunity and complement B cells to produce antibodies. The thymus also produces a variety of thymus hormones that promote the differentiation and maturation of immune lymphocyte stem cells. Although the thymus is a lymphoid organ, due to the presence of the blood thymus barrier, the thymus does not directly interact with the antigen to exert an effect. Thus, it is not proliferated by the stimulation of tumor-specific antigens. The tumor produces secretory immunosuppressive factors that act on the thymus, causing progressive atrophy and functional damage.

About Immunotherapy for malignant tumors many doctors are committed to the development of this field with great interest. As early as 1968, Krant et al reported that the cellular immune function of lung cancer patients was inhibited, and patients had delayed onset of allergic reactions to dinitrochlorobenzene (DNCB) and pure tuberculin (PPD), and found that the body's immune function was affected. The degree of damage increases with the progress of the tumor. In the past 20 years, the relationship between the body's immune status and tumorigenesis, development and prognosis has increasingly attracted the attention of oncologists. Since the 1980s, due to the rapid development of immunology and biotechnology, it has provided an opportunity for immunotherapy for cancer patients. The theory of biological response regulation has been proposed, and a fourth treatment program other than surgery, radiotherapy, and chemotherapy has been established. That is, tumor biotherapy (BRM). The use of biological modulators to treat tumors may be promising for the development of new therapies for effective immunotherapy for tumors.

In short, the host and the tumor are a contradiction, and have existed throughout the process of tumor development and development. When the body's immune system is functioning properly, the body can restrict and destroy the tumor through its cellular and humoral immune responses. On the other hand, the growing tumor has a lot of influence on the body's immune system, inhibiting the body's immune function and promoting the development of the tumor.

6. Animal Discovery Research New Findings 5

Experimental study on the effect of spleen on tumor growth

In recent years, the role of the spleen in anti-tumor immunity has received increasing attention, and its anti-cancer effect is very complicated. There are still many differences and doubts. To further explore the effects of spleen on tumor growth and understand the relationship between spleen and tumor immunity, the Ehrlich ascites model was prepared by experimental surgical method. The spleen group was excised before and after inoculation of cancer cells. The following experiment was performed in comparison with the spleen group to observe the effect of splenectomy on tumor immune status.

【Materials and Methods】

1. The experimental animals were grouped into Kunming mice, which were male or female. The age of the mice was 50' -- '60d, and the weight was 15-20g, a total of 300. According to the spleen and the spleen, the spleen and the inoculated cancer cells were divided into 5 groups according to

different inoculation cells ((1 X 104 ml or 1 X107 ml) and different inoculation sites (abdominal or subcutaneous), each group Divided into subgroups A and B, as shown in Table 1 below.

Table 1 Summary table of experimental animals grouping

Group＼Inoculation Method	cancer cells concentration 1×10^4/ml		cancer cells concentration 1×10^7/ml	
	percutaneous	transabdominal	percutaneous	transabdominal
Group I simulating spleen removal	I A$_1$ (15)	I A$_2$ (15)	I B$_1$ (15)	I B$_2$ (15)
Group II (spleen removal before inoculation)	II A$_1$ (15)	II A$_2$ (15)	II B$_1$ (15)	II B$_2$(15)
Group III (inoculation before spleen removal)	III A (30)		III B (30)	
Group IV (spleen removal before inoculation+ splenic cells)	IV A$_1$ (15)	II A$_2$ (15)	IV B$_1$ (15)	IV B$_2$ (15)
Group V (administration of Chinese medicine)	V A (15)		V B (15)	

Group I: Control group with spleen. Firstly simulating spleen removal, after 7d transabdominal or percutaneous inoculation of Ehrlich ascites cancer cells 0.1ml, the number of cancer cells is 1×10^4 or 1×10^7 (table 2).

Table 2 Control group of simulating spleen removal (Group I)

Group I	Inoculated Cancer Cell Number	Inoculated Regions	Mice Number
I A$_1$	0.1×10^4	right armpit subcutaneousness	15
I A$_2$	0.1×10^4	abdominal cavity	15
I B$_1$	0.1×10^7	right armpit subcutaneousness	15
I B$_2$	0.1×10^7	abdominal cavity	15

Group II: Group of spleen removal before inoculation. Firstly spleen removal, after 7d percutaneous or transabdominal inoculation of Ehrlich ascites cancer cells 0.1ml, the number of cancer cells is 1×10^4 or 1×10^7 (table 3).

Table 3 Group of spleen removal before inoculation

Group II	Inoculated Cancer Cell Number	Inoculated Regions	Mice Number
II A$_1$	0.1×10^4	right armpit subcutaneousness	15
II A$_2$	0.1×10^4	abdominal cavity	15
II B$_1$	0.1×10^7	right armpit subcutaneousness	15
II B$_2$	0.1×10^7	abdominal cavity	15

Group III: Group without spleen, i.e. group of inoculation before spleen removal. Firstly inoculation of cancer cells, after 7d spleen removal. Both are right armpit subcutaneous inoculations. The number of cancer cells is 1×10^4ml or 1×10^7ml (table 4).

Table 4 Group of inoculation before spleen removal

Group III	Inoculated Cancer Cell Number	Inoculated Regions	Mice Number
III A	0.1×10^4	right armpit subcutaneousness	15
III B	0.1×10^7	right armpit subcutaneousness	15

Group IV: Group of spleen removal before inoculation, and further transabdominal transplantation of splenic cells or clear liquid of splenic tissue. Firstly remove spleen, after 7d inoculate cancer cells. In another 1d, transabdominal injection of living spleen cell suspension or supernatant liquid of splenic tissue (table 5).

Table 5 Group of spleen removal before transplantation of splenic cells or clear liquid of splenic tissue

Group IV	Inoculated Cancer Cell Number	Inoculated Regions	Processing Factor	Mice Number
IV A$_1$	0.1×10^4	trans-sub right armpit	injection of supernatant liquid of splenic tissue	15
IV A$_2$	0.1×10^4	transabdominal	injection of supernatant liquid of splenic tissue	15
IV B$_1$	0.1×10^7	right armpit subcutaneousness	transplantation of splenic cells of newborn mice	15
IV B$_2$	0.1×10^7	abdominal cavity	transplantation of splenic cells of adult mice	15

Group V: Group of taking Traditional Chinese Medicine (TCM) complex prescription with efficacy of strengthening the spleen and replenishing qi (table 6).

Table 6 Group of taking Traditional Chinese Medicine (TCM) complex prescription with efficacy of strengthening the spleen and replenishing qi

Group V	Inoculated Cancer Cell Number	Inoculated Regions	Processing Factor	Mice Number
V A	$10^7 \times 0.1$	right armpit subcutaneousness	firstly take TCM for 10d, after inoculation continue to take medication for 3 weeks	15
V B	$10^7 \times 0.1$	right armpit subcutaneousness	after inoculation take medication for 3 weeks	15

2. Instruments and Materials

(1) An animal sterile operating room and a set of sterile surgical instruments.

(2) Hank liquid, improved Hank liquid, calf serum, PRH, triple-distilled water, 0.9% sodium chloride solution for injection, ketamine, soluble phenobarbital, heparin sodium, trypan blue stain, Giemsa stain, Wright's stain, hydrochloric acid baking soda, L-glutamic acid, sensitization and non- sensitization zymosan.

(3) Centrifugal machine with 400 rounds per minute, glass homogenizer, medicine vibrator, filtering metal gauze (size 1000), funnel, thermostat, baker, low temperature water tank, microscope, relative sterile workbench.

(4) Animal feed are refined pellet feed. The drinking water is tap water. Rearing cage is plastic mouse cage.

3. Tumor Inoculation and Model Preparation

Ehrlich ascites tumor cell strain is introduced from Wuhan Biological Research Institute Cell Room. Ascites containing cancer cells are extracted from ascetic-type tumor animal abdominal cavity of mice Ehrlich ascites tumor. Firstly use improved Hank liquid to clean and centrifugate ascites for 3 times with 800 rounds per minute of centrifugal speed and five minutes. Remove supernatant liquid, and respectively combine deposited cancer cells with Hank liquid to make up the cancer cell suspensions, containing 1×10^4 ml or 1×10^7 ml inoculated cells. The trypan blue dead cells exclusion test proves that the living cell rate is above 95%. Then inoculate cancer cells to experimental mice through right armpit subcutaneousness and abdominal cavity. Each mouse is inoculated with cancer cell suspension of 0.1ml, i.e. amounts of containing cancer cells are 1×10^4 ml or 1×10^7 ml.

4. Splenectomy

Combine ketamine with soluble phenobarbital to execute intraperitoneal anesthesia. Dosages are 0.4mg/10g and 0.2mg/10g. After anesthesia, fix the mouse on surgery board. Shear the belly fur. Use iodine (2.5%) and ethanol (75%) to disinfect the belly. Bespread the sterile cloth on it. An incision is made into each layer of abdominal wall tissue through left lower abdomen. Then enter into abdominal cavity. Expose and dissociate the spleen. Use silk thread of size 0 to ligate the splenic stalk. Excise the spleen. Ensure the strict sterile operation, gentle action and thorough hemostases. During the operation, notice whether there is a splenulus. In case there is, excise it together. For simulating spleen removal of control group, only open the abdominal cavity; pull but do not excise the spleen. Antibiotics are not used in and after the operation. Infection of incisional wound is 1.0%. After operation, continue to feed the mouse with refined pellet feed.

5. Preparations of Splenic Cell Suspension and Supernatant Liquid of Splenic Tissue

(1) Preparation of splenic cell suspension: Execute newborn Kunming mice of 24-48h or adult mice. An incision is made into abdominal wall to take out the spleen. Cut off peripheral envelope and adipose tissue of spleen. Use Hank liquid to irrigate them in sterile glass culture dish for 3 times. Then put spleen into the glass homogenizer. Add in Hank liquid for 5ml. Grind up the splenic tissue. Filter it with stainless silk net of size 100. Centrifugate the filtering medium (1000 rounds per minute, 10 min). Remove supernatant liquid. Use Hank liquid to dilute deposited cells and make up the splenic cell suspensions of 5×10^7/ml. Suspensions are dyed by trypan blue stain and proved that the living cell rate is above 97%. Then transplant splenic cell suspensions into abdominal cavity of experimental mouse. Each mouse can only accept splenic cell suspensions of 2ml which belong to one receptor.

(2) Preparation of splenic cell homogenate: After excising the spleen, use quick freezing (-20 centi degree) and rapid rewarming to induce the cracking of dead splenic cells proved by trypan blue stain and microscopic examination. Then centrifugate the filtering medium (1000 rounds per minute, 10 min). Reserve supernatant liquid and remove deposits. Inject supernatant liquid through abdomen into the experimental mouse.

6. Observation Item

(1) Observe success ratio of cancer cell inoculation, occurrence time of subcutaneous tumor nodi and speed of tumor enlargement.

(2) Every day use vernier caliper to measure diameter and size of subcutaneous tumor nodi; measure mouse' weight; observe metastasis condition and moving degree.

(3) Observe the quality of life, fur color, vitality, state of nutrition, breath, mental state of tumor-bearing mice and survival time of bearing tumor.

(4) Observe abdominal shape and prohection of ascetic-type tumor-bearing mice. Also according to prohection state, divide ascites content into 5 grades.

Grade 0: the abdomen is not of fullness, without ascites, note as (-).

Grade 1: slight prohection of abdomen, with a little ascites, note as (+).

Grade 2: prohection of abdomen, with medium content of ascites, note as (++).

Grade 3: obvious prohection of abdomen, with more ascites, note as (+++).

Grade 4: shape of frog abdomen, with plentiful ascites, note as (++++).

During necropsy, measure the content of ascites, microscopic examination of cancer cell shape, count living cell rate and content.

(5) Determine immunologic functional condition of red blood cells of tumor-bearing mice: test for measuring C_3b receptor garland with semi quantitative method.

(6) Necropsy and pathological section: dissect each dead experimental mouse. Observe tumor's size and weight, infiltrating and metastatic condition, morphological structure and involvement condition of visceral organs; measure the content of ascites; extract tumor tissue, liver, spleen, thymus gland, lung and other visceral organs to carry out the examination of pathological section.

[Experimental Result]

1. Resulting comparison and analysis on different groups with right armpit subcutaneous inoculation of small dose of 0.1×10^4 ml Ehrlich ascites tumor cells.

(1) Comparison on occurrence time of tumor nodi with different processing method (T test), see table 7.

Table 7 Comparison on occurrence time (d) of tumor nodi with different processing method (T test)

Group	Group I A_1	Group II A_1	Group IIIA	Group IVA$_1$
	(Control group with spleen)	(Group of spleen removal before inoculation)	(Group of inoculation before spleen removal)	(Spleen removal before inoculation+supernatant liquid of splenic tissue)
Occurrence time (d)	8	7*	9	9*

Note: ① *. Compared with Group I A_1, P<0.05 has remarkable significance; ② In Group I A_1 (control group with spleen), one experimental mouse (accounts for 7.6%) suffers no tumor nodi after inoculation of cancer cells. It survives for a long term (i.e. survival time is above 90d). No tumor is found during dissection. Treat it as inoculation failure. Not for statistical treatment;

also in Group IVA (group with transabdominal injection of supernatant liquid of splenic tissue), 3 experimental mice (accounts for 25%) fail to be inoculated.

According to table 7, the earliest occurrence time of tumor nodi in above groups belongs to group of spleen removal before inoculation (Group II A$_1$). Control group and group with injection of supernatant liquid of splenic tissue have the later occurrence time.

(2) For different processing methods, maximum diameter comparison of each group's tumor nodi on the seventh, fourteenth and twentieth day, see table 8.

Table 8 Size comparison of each group's tumor nodi on the seventh, fourteenth and twentieth day after subcutaneous inoculation of 0.1×10^4 ml cancer cells (maximum diameter mm)

Group	Group I A$_1$	Group II A$_1$	Group III A	Group IVA$_1$	P
	(Control group with spleen)	(Group of spleen removal before inoculation)	(Group of inoculation before spleen removal)	(Spleen removal before inoculation+supernatant liquid of splenic tissue)	
seventh	0	3.3±0.48	0	0	<0.01
fourteenth	11.43±5.99	14.4±6.2	11.8±7.45	8±4.33	<0.01
twentieth	18.92±9.98	21.12±8.28	19.7±5.98	13.89±7.63	<0.01

Note: Values *P* in the table are gained through analysis of diameter variance (*F* test).

From above results in the table, the tumor which belongs to group of spleen removal before inoculation (Group II A$_1$) appears first and grows fast. Before the fourteenth day, its tumor volume reaches biggest. On the twentieth day after inoculation, tumors' sizes of control group (Group I A$_1$), group II A$_1$ (group of spleen removal before inoculation), group of inoculation before spleen removal (Group III A) reach unanimity. While tumors which belong to group of injecting supernatant liquid of splenic tissue (Group IV A$_1$) have the smallest volume. That explains that during early growing stage of tumor (before the seventh day), spleen has tumor inhibitory action. But during medium and advanced stages (experimental group sets: medium stage is from eighth day to fourteenth day since the inoculation; since the fourteenth day, it is tumor advanced stage), the inhibitory action of spleen weakens or disappears. Furthermore, it can be observed that after cancer cells inoculation of spleen removal group, since the fourteenth day, tumor nodi often bear liquefaction, necrosis and ablation, which result in the shrinkage of tumor volume. Even some incisions have healed. Why does such phenomenon appear? That needs to have a further observation.

(3) Comparison of mean survival time (MST) for groups of subcutaneous inoculation with 0.1×10^4 ml cancer cells, see table 9.

Table 9 Comparison of each group's mean survival time (MST)

Group	Group I A$_1$ (Control group with spleen)	Group II A$_1$ (Group of spleen removal before inoculation)	Group III A (Group of inoculation before spleen removal)	Group IVA$_1$ (Spleen removal before inoculation＋supernatant liquid of splenic tissue)	P
MST (d)	41.61±12.24	38.73±19.63	44.8±15.95	50±27.21	<0.05

Note: Values *P* in the table are gained through *F* test.

From table 9, mean survival times of groups I A$_1$, II A$_1$, III A are close to each other. T test shows there is no difference among these three groups, *P* > 0.05. While for injection of supernatant liquid of splenic tissue, mean survival time of this group is obviously longer than those of other groups, *P* < 0.05. The significant difference exists.

2. Resulting analysis of each group's transabdominal inoculation with 0.1×10^4 ml cancer cells
After inoculation of cancer cells, experimental mice can survive above 90d without any ascite or tumor nodus. Also a dissection of corpse shows no tumor. The above results are treated as inoculation failures. It explains the fact that vaccinal cancer cells are rejected by the organism and no tumor forms.

(1) Comparison of inoculation failure rate for each group's transabdominal inoculation of 0.1×10^4 ml cancer cells without ascites, see table 10.

Table 10 Comparison of each group's inoculation failure rate (T test)

Group	Group I A$_2$ (Control group with spleen)	Group II A$_2$ (Group of spleen removal before inoculation)	Group II A$_2$ (Spleen removal before inoculation＋supernatant liquid of splenic tissue)
failure rate	26%	0**	54%*

Note: **. indicates the comparison with control group, T test *P*<0.01, with high degree of significant difference; *. indicates *P*<0.05, with significant difference.

Results of table 10 show that all experimental mice in the group of spleen removal before inoculation form ascites, and failure rate is zero. The inoculation failure rates of control group with spleen and injection group of supernatant liquid of splenic tissue are 26% and 54% respectively. It process that tumor is easy to grow in the mouse without spleen after inoculation of tumor. That is, the removal of spleen promotes the growth of tumor. On the contrary, injection of supernatant liquid of splenic cells will suppress the growth of tumor.

(2) Comparison of survival time for each group's transabdominal inoculation of 0.1×10^4 ml cancer cells, see table 11.

Table 11 Comparison of each group's survival time (F test)

Group	Group I A$_2$ (Control group with spleen)	Group II A$_2$ (Group of spleen removal before inoculation)	Group IVA$_2$ (Spleen removal before inoculation+supernatant liquid of splenic tissue)	P
survival time (d)	51.46±29.35	35.6±18.93	57.6±14.85	<0.05

From table 11, the mean survival time of group with spleen removal before inoculation is 35.6±18.93 days. While mean survival times of control group with spleen and injection group of supernatant liquid of splenic tissue are 51.46±29.35 days and 57.6±14.85 days respectively, and P<0.05. Significant differences exist among these three groups. In three groups, group of spleen removal before inoculation has the shortest survival time. Group with spleen owns long survival time; while group without spleen owns short survival time. That shows the removal of spleen promotes the growth of tumor and shortens survival times of tumor-bearing mice. On the contrary, injection of supernatant liquid of splenic cells will suppress the growth of tumor and prolong survival times of tumor-bearing mice.

3. Results of each group's subcutaneous inoculation with 0.1×10^7 ml cancer cells

(1) Comparison on occurrence time of each group's subcutaneous tumor nodi, see table 12.

Table 12 Comparison on occurrence time of each group's subcutaneous tumor nodi

Group	Group I B$_1$ (Control group with spleen)	Group II B$_1$ (Group of spleen removal before inoculation)	Group III B (Group of inoculation before spleen removal)	Group IV B$_1$ (Spleen removal before inoculation+transplantation of fetal mouse's splenic cells)	P
Occurrence time (d)	5.5	5	7.5	9	<0.05

Mice of group IIIB are removed spleens on the seventh day after inoculations. So after seven days group IIIB and control group with spleen (Group I B₁) are in the same condition. The table shows that for the group with spleen removal first, occurrence times of subcutaneous tumor nodi are slightly earlier than these of other groups. While for group IVB₁ (transplantation of fetal mouse's splenic cells), occurrence times of tumor nodi are obviously later than these of other groups. It proves that the removal of spleen promotes the growth of tumor. While transplantation of splenic cells intensively suppresses the growth of tumor.

(2) Comparison of maximum diameter average on each group's subcutaneous tumor nodi on the seventh, fourteenth and twentieth day after inoculation, see table 13.

Table 13 Comparison of maximum diameter on each group's tumor nodi on the seventh, fourteenth and twentieth day (mm)

Group	Group I B1 (Control group with spleen)	Group II B1 (Group of spleen removal before inoculation)	Group III B (Group of inoculation before spleen removal)	Group IV B1 (Spleen removal before inoculation+transplantation of fetal mouse's splenic cells)	P
seventh	5.07±1.847	10.88±5.278	2.83±1.948	3.0±1.56	<0.01
fourteenth	19.85±4.598	21.12±5.3	20.3±6.07	11±5.69	<0.01
twentieth	30.9±7.87	24±7.86	25.25±4.77	16±4.95	<0.01

Note: Values P in the table are gained through F test.

(3) Comparison of each group's mean survival time (MST), see table 22-14.

Table 14 Comparison of each group's mean survival time (subcutaneous inoculation of $0.1×10^7$ ml cancer cells)

Group	Group I B₁ (Control group with spleen)	Group II B₁ (Group of spleen removal before inoculation)	Group III B	Group IV B₁ (Spleen removal before inoculation+transplantation of fetal mouse's splenic cells)	P
MST (d)	33.1±13.15	49.56±24.39	38.7±14.45	50.75±19.30	<0.01

From table 13 and 14, on the seventh day after inoculation, for the three groups-control group with spleen (Group IB_1), group of spleen removal before inoculation (Group IIB_1) and group of inoculation before spleen removal (Group IIIB), their maximum diameter averages of tumor nodi are $\overline{X}(IB_1) = (5.07\pm1.847)$ mm, $\overline{X}(IIB_1) = (10.88\pm5.278)$ mm, $\overline{X}(IIIB) = (2.83\pm1.948)$ mm respectively. *P*<0.01. Significant differences exist among these three groups. Tumors which belong to the group of spleen removal before inoculation (IIB_1) have the maximum volumes. Now on the seventh day, in fact groups IB_1 and IIIB have the spleen, which is in proliferative active phase. While group IIB_1 has no spleen. The tumor volume of group with spleen is smaller, and the tumor volume of group without spleen is larger. It indicates that the spleen can suppress tumor during early stage or the removal of spleen can promote the growth of tumor. While on the fourteenth day after inoculation, their average maximum diameters of tumor nodi are $\overline{X}(IB_1) = (19.85\pm4.598)$ mm, $\overline{X}(IIB_1) = (21.12\pm5.3)$ mm, $\overline{X}(IIIB) = (20.3\pm6.07)$ mm respectively. *P*>0.05. Significant differences disappear among these three groups. On the twentieth day after inoculation, the tumor volume of control group with spleen is larger than that of other groups. The maximum diameter $\overline{X} = (30.9\pm7.87)$ mm. At this time, the spleen of tumor-bearing mouse has extremely shrank, and lost the tumor inhibitory action. From the experiment, since the fourteenth day after inoculation, most mice tumors of group with spleen removal begin to bear liquefaction and necrosis. Some lumps ulcerate and ablate, whose volumes shrink. The reason that tumors in this period suffer from liquefaction, necrosis and ulceration is not clear at present. That needs to have a further observation.

Therefore, during the early stage of tumor, spleen can suppress the growth of tumor. For the group with spleen, the tumor growth rate is slower. Tumor volume is smaller. While on the advanced stage of tumor, the inhibitory action of spleen weakens or disappears. The tumor size of all groups reaches unanimity.

Furthermore, it can be seen from the stable that tumors of the group (IVB_1), which removes spleen before inoculation and transplants splenic cells of fetal mice, have obviously slower growth rate than that of other groups. The tumor volume is smaller. Its survival time is longer that that of other groups. These conditions prove that splenic cells of homogeneous variant fetus have obvious tumor-inhibitory action.

4. Results of each group's transabdominal inoculation with 0.1×10^7 ml cancer cells

   (1)   Comparison on occurrence time of ascites for each group, see table 22-15.

Table 15 Comparison on occurrence time of ascites for each group of transabdominal inoculation with 0.1×10⁷ ml cancer cells

Group	Group I B$_2$	Group II B$_2$	Group IV B$_2$
	(Control group with spleen)	(Group of spleen removal before inoculation)	(Spleen removal before inoculation+transplantation of splenic cells)
Occurrence time (median, d)	5	3*	4*

Note: **. indicates the comparison with control group, T test *P*<0.05, with significant difference.

(2) Occupying percentages of ascites content greater than (++) for groups on the fifth, seventh and fourteenth day after transabdominal inoculation of 0.1×10⁷ ml cancer cells, see table 16.

Table 16 Comparison on ascites content of transabdominal inoculation with 0.1×10⁷ ml cancer cells

Days after inoculation (d)	Group I B$_2$	Group II B$_2$	Group IV B$_2$
	(Control group with spleen)	(Group of spleen removal before inoculation)	(Spleen removal before inoculation+transplantation of splenic cells)
2	0%	75% **	10% *
7	28%	100% **	70% *
14	100%	100%	100% *

Note: **. indicates the comparison with IB$_2$ (control group), T test *P*<0.01; *. indicates *P*<0.05; no *. indicates *P*>0.05.

(3) Comparison of survival time (d) for each group's transabdominal inoculation of 0.1×10⁷ ml cancer cells, see table 17.

Table 17 Comparison of each group's survival time

Group	Group I B$_2$	Group II B$_2$	Group IV B$_2$
	(Control group with spleen)	(Group of spleen removal before inoculation)	(Spleen removal before inoculation+transplantation of splenic cells)
survival time (d)	20.15±4.59	15.56±10.94*	16.67±8.34

Note: *. indicates the comparison with IB$_2$, *P*<0.05, with significant difference; no *. indicates the comparison with IB$_2$, *P*>0.05, without significant difference.

Integrating tables 15, 16 and 17, results show that for the group with spleen removal first (IIB$_2$), tumor growth rate is faster. Amounts of ascites are more. Survival time is shorter. Also visceral organs are easier to metastasize. Those explain that removal of spleen can promote the growth of tumor. Transabdominal transplantation of splenic cells of homogeneous variant adult mice can partially suppress the growth of tumor. But its inhibitory action is weaker than that of control group with spleen and group with transplantation of fetal mouse's splenic cells.

5. Results of necropsy and pathological examination Each mouse accepts the postmortem necropsy. Visually observe tumor shape, involved visceral organs and diffusion condition. And extract tissues for pathological section examination. The result shows that Ehrlich ascites tumor cell strain owns features of stable proliferation, strong invasiveness and so on. Subcutaneous inoculation is easy to induce the form of solid tumor. Necropsy proves that after inoculation tumors or ascites are easy to form in some regions, easily infiltrating to surrounding tissues. The metastases of cancer cells rarely happen to mice with subcutaneous inoculation. While for mice with transabdominal inoculation, cancer cells easily metastasize to liver, kidney and lymph node in advanced stage. Only two of two hundred and seventy experimental mice suffer from splenic metastases, proving the weak affinity of spleen to cancer cells. This group of experiments has also found phenomena that for the group of spleen removal before transabdominal inoculation, multiple carcinomatous metastases appear in visceral organs of abdominal cavity. Metastatic ratio is up to 50%. These metastases invade liver, kidney, pancreas and mesenteric lymph nodes, always implicating more than two visceral organs. While for control group with spleen and group with transplantation of homogeneous variant splenic cells, carcinomatous metastases rarely occur. Metastatic ratios are 20% and 25%, which are obviously lower than those of the group without spleen. It shows that spleen can suppress the growth of tumor. While the group without spleens lose the inhibitory action, consequently leading to easy diffusion and metastasis of tumor.

Furthermore, dynamic observation of this group of experimental mice shows that thymus and spleen of tumor-bearing mice present a series of changes with the process of illness, which own certain regularity. About seven days after inoculation, the thymus presents acute and progressive atrophy. Its volume shrinks; the diameter of each normal lobule shortens from 5~8cm to about 1mm; the weight reduces from (70±10) mg to (20±5) mg. While soon after the inoculation of cancer cells, spleen becomes congested and tumid. The volume enlarges; weight increases; texture becomes fragile. Microscopic examination shows the increase of germinal centers and active cell proliferation. On the fourteenth day after inoculation, the spleen also quickly presents progressive atrophy. Its volume shrinks; the weight reduces from (140±15) mg to (50±10) mg. Germinal centers obviously decrease; cell proliferation is suffocated. The spleen also suffers from hyperplasia of fibrous tissues, fibrosis with gray color and rigid texture.

6. Testing results of erythrocytic immune function This group of experiments choose 100 mice to carry out the erythrocytic C_3b receptor garland test. The result shows that after the removal of spleen, bonding ratio of C_3b receptor garland of tumor-bearing mice is on a progressive declining tendency. That explains that after the removal of spleen, immunological adhesive competence of red blood cells drops to some extent.

[Discussion]

1. As seen from experimental results, spleen can suppress the growth of tumor.

After the removal of spleen, compared with the control group, the growth rate is faster; the occurrence time and volume of subcutaneous tumor nodi is earlier and larger in the same period. For group with transabdominal inoculation of cancer cells and group with the removal of spleen, occurrence time of ascites is earlier; ascites content is greater; cells content is also higher. Survival time is shorter than that of control group. Necropsy finds that cancer metastatic rate of the group with the removal of spleen is 30% above that of control group (metastases to liver, kidney, pancreas and mesenteric lymph nodes). From table 13, group IIB_1 (spleen removal before inoculation) and group IIIB (inoculation before spleen removal) accept splenectomy in different time. On the seventh day after inoculation, maximum diameter averages of their subcutaneous tumor nodi are $\overline{X}(IIB_1)$ = (10.8±5.28) mm and $\overline{X}(IIIB)$ = (2.83±1.948) mm respectively. The former is obviously longer than the latter one. But on the fourteenth day after inoculation, the tumor of group IIIB quickly proliferates after the removal of spleen. The difference between them almost disappears. $\overline{X}(IIB_1)$ = (21.2±5.3) mm, $\overline{X}(IIIB)$ = (20.3±6.07), $P>0.05$, without significant difference. It prompts that the removal of spleen promotes the growth of tumor, i.e. spleen can suppress the growth of tumor.

In recent two decades, people find **that spleen not only performs a great role in anti-infection, but also has the all-important influence on anti-tumor immunity**. The active mechanism may be by producing Natural Killer cell, macrophage (MΦ), Lympholine-Activated Killer cell, TH/Ti cell, B cell, Ts cell, etc. to realize the cellular immunity; and by secreting lymphokines of Tufisn factor, TNF factor, IL-2, interferon, addiment, antibody, etc. to kill tumor cells. Ge Yigong once used rat Lw56 pulmonary sarcoma model to the effect of removing spleen on tumor growth. Mr Ge holds that success ratio of tumor inoculation after the removal of spleen is higher than that of group with spleen. The metastatic ratio increases. Results are similar to this group of experimental results.

This group of experimental results also prompts that after the removal of spleen, bonding ratio of C_3b receptor garland of organism peripheral blood is 40% below that of healthy group with spleen. It explains that erythrocytic immune function of organism reduces after the removal of spleen.

2. Spleen's inhibiting action on tumor growth mainly occurs in the early stage of tumor course. While in the advanced stage of tumor, spleen's inhibiting action on tumor growth weakens and disappears.

As seen from tables 8 and 13, in the early stage of tumor (within 7d), the tumor of group without spleen has a faster tumor growth rate than that of control group with spleen. The volume of subcutaneous tumor nodi is large and ascites content is great. While in the advanced stage (after 14d) of tumor, tumor nodi of control group with spleen and group with the removal of spleen basically have the same volume. No significant comparability. No obvious difference between survival times. Necropsy and pathological examination of three hundred experimental mice find that spleen of tumor-bearing mice present a series of regular changes with the process of illness. In the early stage of tumor (within 7d after inoculation), due to the cytostimulation, the spleen becomes congested and tumid. The volume enlarges; cell proliferation accelerates; germinal centers increases. While in the advanced stage (since 14d after inoculation) of tumor, the spleen presents progressive atrophy. Its volume shrinks; germinal centers fall sharply. The spleen also suffers from hyperplasia of fibrous tissues. The fibrosis of spleen occurs; therefore, its anticancer immunization weakens or disappears. Even it can pass through the suppressor T cell. Macrophage and immune inhibiting factor can suppress the anticancer immunization of organism and promote the growth of tumor. That explains that spleen's effect on tumor immune state is bidirectional, has obvious time phase and is relevant to stadium. In early stage, the spleen owns the anti-tumor action. In advanced stage, the spleen owns immune inhibiting action. But the basic reason that leads to the immune inhibiting state of organism is the tumor itself. Spleen just plays a certain part in the forming process of this state.

3. Transabdominal injection of supernatant liquid of healthy splenic cells and transplantation of homogeneous variant splenic cells can suppress tumor growth.

For group of injection with supernatant liquid of splenic cells or transplantation of splenic cells (Group IV), comparative results with other groups show that the tumor growth rate is slower; the occurrence time of tumor nodi is later; the volume is smaller; ascites content is less. After the inoculation of small dose of 0.1×10^4 ml cancer cells, success ratio of inoculation for tumor-bearing mice is obviously lower than that of other groups. Moreover, after a little ascites or subcutaneous lesser tubercle firstly appearing in several mice, the tumor can disappear naturally. The survival time is above 90d (as long-term survivors). Especially splenic cells of homogeneous variant fetal mouse (group IVB_1) have obvious tumor-inhibitory action. The tumor inhibition rate is 54%.

The survival time is 17d longer than that of control group. Pathological examinations of this group of tumor-bearing mice find that after transplantation of homogeneous variant fetal splenic cells, splenic islands grow on the abdominal cavity and (or) mesentery of seven mice (account for 50%). Pathological examination proves it as living splenic tissues. Fetal splenic cells have features of weak antigenicity, deficient quantity and strong cell proliferation, etc. After the transplantation of splenic cells of homogeneous variant mice, there is no sharp rejection. And moreover, it is not subject to blood group ABO. Do notneed the cross test of different blood groups. Here in China some people use traumatic splenic cells to prepare LAK cells for treating advanced malignant tumors, which achieves better curative effects on inhibiting tumor growth and prolonging mouse's lifespan.

At present, adoptive immunotherapy of tumors with transplantation of fetal splenic cells has not yet been reported in the literature. This group of experiments needs to have a further observation.

4. Negative correlation between anti-tumor immunological action of the organism and the quantity of cancer cells

This group of experiments finds that anti-tumor immunological action of the organism is obviously affected by the quantity of inoculated cancer cells. The less the quantity of cancer cells, the stronger and more significant the anti-tumor effect; on the contrary, the weaker the anti-tumor effect. As for 0.1×10^7 ml inoculated cancer cells, immunological action of the organism is obviously suppressed. The tumor growth rates of group without spleen and group with spleen have bigger difference in the early stage. While after medium stage (after 7d), the difference will quickly disappear. There is also no significant difference in survival time. But for 0.1×10^4 ml inoculated cancer cells, anti-tumor action of the organism is relatively significant. The inoculated failure rate of group with spleen is obviously higher than that of group without spleen. The growth rate of tumor is slow; the volume of tumor nodi is small; and the survival time is long. Furthermore, after the transplantation of homogeneous variant splenic cells for small dose of inoculated cancer cells group, anti-tumor immunological action goes up remarkably. The growth rate of tumor decreases obviously. Some tumor nodi even can naturally disappear after its formation. Also the survival time is long. These results show the negative correlation between anti-tumor action of the organism and the quantity of inoculated cancer cells. While there is a positive correlation between cancer's immunological inhibiting action on the organism and the quantity of inoculated cancer cells. The spleen participates in tumor immunoregulation, which has double influences on immune state of tumor-bearing mice. In early stage, the spleen shows a certain anti-cancer action. As the development of tumor, the number of tumor cells is increasing. The spleen is shrinking gradually. Then the anti-cancer action is converted into immunological inhibiting action. But the basic reason of immune inhibiting state is the tumor itself. The progress of cancer, an increase in the number of cancer cells and the reinforcement of inhibiting action lead to the atrophia of spleen, thymus gland and other immune organs.

5. Experimental result prompts of this group

(1) The spleen has certain anti-tumor effects. In tumor's early stage, spleen can suppress the growth of tumor. While in advanced stage of the course of disease, the anti-tumor action of spleen weakens or disappears. The spleen even can promote the growth of spleen.

(2) Adoptive immunotherapy of tumors with transplantation of homogeneous variant splenic cells of fetal mice can reinforce anti-tumor immunological action of the organism, and suppress the growth of tumor.

(3) There is a negative correlation between anti-tumor action of the organism and the quantity of inoculated cancer cells. The more the quantity of cancer cells, the more easily the immunological action of the organism is suppressed or damaged. The faster the growth rate of tumor, the worse the prognosis.

7. New Discovery of Animal Experiment Research 6:

Experimental study on anti-tumor and immune enhancement of traditional Chinese medications with supporting righness and firming the body

1. Drugs that improve immune function should be used in advanced cancer treatment.

1). The discovery of tumor real face research

In the late stage of cancer, the mice have low immune function and progressive atrophy of the thymus. When the author's laboratory conducts experiments on the production of tumor-bearing animal models, the thymus can be removed to produce a tumor-bearing animal model, and it is difficult to manufacture an animal model without removing the thymus. The results of the study demonstrate that there is a clear positive relationship between the occurrence and development of cancer and the host's immune function and thymus function.

Whether it is first immune system is low and then easy to get cancer, or cancer first and then immune function is low, the author's experimental results are low immunity and then easy to have cancer, if no immune function decline, it is not easy to vaccinate successfully. The results of this study suggest that improving and maintaining good immune function and protecting the immune organs thymus are one of the important measures to prevent cancer.

In the author's laboratory, the animal model of liver metastasis was established when the relationship between cancer metastasis and immunity was divided into A and B groups. Group A used immunosuppressive drugs, and group B did not. As a result, the number of intrahepatic metastases in group A was significantly higher than that in group B. The results of this experiment suggest that metastasis is associated with immunity, low immune function or the use of immunosuppressive drugs to promote tumor metastasis.

In the experiment of the effect of tumor on the immune organs of the body, it was found that as the cancer progressed, the thymus was inhibited by progressive cell proliferation and the volume was significantly reduced. The results of this experiment suggest that the tumor will inhibit the thymus and cause the immune organs to shrink.

The above experimental results show that the occurrence, development and metastasis of cancer are significantly related to the decline of immune function of the host. The advanced cancer in mice has low immune function and progressive atrophy of the thymus. Therefore, in the treatment of advanced cancer, drugs that improve immune function should be used, and drugs that reduce or suppress immunity should not be used.

2). To find ways to improve immune function and inhibit tumors from natural medicines

In order to stop the atrophy of immune organs when tumors progress, to find ways to restore thymus function and make immune reconstruction, the author began to look for anti-cancer drugs that enhance high immune function from natural drugs. . After long-term and batch-wise screening of 200 kinds of traditional anti-cancer Chinese herbal medicines, the tumor-inhibiting screening experiments in tumor-bearing animals were carried out. The results showed that 152 kinds were ineffective, and only 48 kinds had certain or even better anti-cancer effects. It has the effect of increasing immunity. Among them, 26 kinds of Chinese herbal medicines also have the effect of enhancing macrophage function or stimulating the thymus of animal immune organs to increase or increase white blood cells; or promoting spleen lymphocyte proliferation, increasing lymphocyte transformation rate and enhancing T cells and enhance the role of immune function, enhance the activity of NK cells, promote the inducing effect of interferon, and optimize the combination, and then in vivo anti-tumor experiments in liver cancer, gastric cancer, S180 and other tumor-bearing animal models, further screen and eliminate the combinations with stability effects, further screening before the composition of xz-c immunomodulation and anti-cancer Chinese medicine, can protect the thymus and increase the immune function, protect the marrow hematopoietic function, improve immune function. Based on the successful screening of animal experiments, it has been applied in clinical practice. After 35 years of clinical verification of a large number of cases, xz-c immunomodulation of traditional Chinese medicine can improve the quality of life of patients with advanced cancer, increase immunity, enhance physical fitness, and improve appetite and to prolong survival and the effect is more significant.

2. Experimental study on the anti-tumor and immune enhancement with Chinese medications of supporting rightness and firming the body system on S 180 mice

1). purpose

Through more than 60 years of research and practice on the prevention and treatment of malignant tumors by Chinese and Western medicine in China, it has been found that many Chinese medicines have certain curative effects on the treatment of tumors, especially the traditional Chinese medicines with the effect of strengthening the right to cure the tumors. This class of traditional Chinese medicine can enhance physical fitness, improve human immune function, improve quality of life and prolong survival. However, most of my treatments for cancer are clinical experience observations, but no experimental studies have been conducted. In order to explore whether the traditional Chinese medicine Fuzheng Pei's spleen, Yiqi Yangxue and Bushen Chinese medicine can inhibit tumor growth, a series of experimental studies were carried out.

2). Method

(1) Experimental animals: 160 Kunming mice, 5---6 weeks old, weighing (27 ± 2.0) g, male and female.

(2) Tumor-bearing animal model:

S-1180 ascites strains were inoculated subcutaneously into the right forelimb axilla of each experimental rat according to 1xi0, pc/ml, and 0.2 rr.

(3) Experimental grouping:

The experimental animals were randomly divided into the following groups.
Group A: Buzhong Yiqi treatment group (n=20).
Group B: qi and blood double-treatment group (n=20),
Group C: nourishing kidney and yin treatment group (n=20)
Group D: Wenbu Shenyang treatment group (n=20)
Group E: ATCA mixture treatment group ((n=20).
Group F: Xiaochaihu Tang treatment group ((n=20),
Group G: Compound capsule treatment group (n=20).
Group H: tumor-bearing control group (n=20),

The groups were started on the 2nd day after inoculation, and were administered with Chinese herbal medicines at 0. 4ml/(d·d) respectively. The tumor-bearing control group was treated with the same amount of physiological saline.

(4) Preparation of traditional Chinese medicines in each group:

It is made into a modern dose of boiling and concentrated according to the original side, and the concentration of the crude drug is 200 rings. The seven drug concentrations and the gavage dose were obtained by replacing the normal human dose with the mouse dose.

In this experiment, Fuzhong Pei Ben›s Buzhong Yiqi, Qi and blood double supplement, nourishing kidney yin, warming kidney yang, attacking and applying ATCA mixture, Xiaochaihu decoction and compound capsule were used to treat S-180 mice.

(5) Observation project:

The tumor appearance time and tumor-bearing survival time of each group of mice were systematically observed, and their serum protein content, peripheral blood T lymphocyte count and weight of immune organs were measured.

3). result

The combination of Fuzheng Peiben and Fuzheng Pei Ben as the main component of ATCA mixture can significantly delay the tumor emergence time and inhibit tumor growth (ABC, D, E group inhibition rate were 40%, 45%, 44.5%, respectively). .31% and 36%), prolonging the survival time of tumor-bearing mice (A, B, C, D, E survival prolongation were 27.6%, 45%, 38.5%, 25% and 26.5%)).

Xiaochaihu Decoction and Compound Capsules, which are mainly based on cockroaches, can not significantly inhibit tumor growth and prolong survival ($P>0.05$ compared with group E). The serum protein content of group A, B, C, D and E increases, A The ratio of /C increased, and the peripheral blood T lymphocyte count increased ($P<0.05$ compared with group C, $P<0.01$) in group B and C, and thymus atrophy was significantly inhibited.

4). Conclusion

Wood research indicates that Fuzheng Peiben or traditional Chinese medicine treatment based on Fuzheng Pei Ben can inhibit tumors and enhance immunity, and can increase the level of peripheral blood T lymphocytes in different degrees, which is more effective than treatment based on phlegm.

5). discuss

(1) The effect of Anti-tumor and prolonging survival with the treatment of Chinese medications of supporting rightness and firm the body system function:

Many cancer patients can clinically show "virtual or false" symptoms, such as qi deficiency, blood deficiency, yin deficiency, and yang deficiency. Treatment should be treated with chinese medications of supporting rightness and firm the body system function. This experiment explored the anti-tumor effect of the various methods of supporting rightness and firming the body system function and the combination of attack and compensation. The results showed that Buzhong Yiqi, Qi and blood double supplement, nourishing kidney yin warming kidney yang and other Fuzheng Peiben traditional Chinese medicine and Fuzheng Peiben traditional Chinese medicine treatment The main ATCA mixture can significantly delay the time of tumor inoculation in mice, inhibit tumor growth, and prolong the survival of tumor-bearing mice. From the analysis of the inhibition rate of each group, the inhibition rate of the qi and blood double-compound experimental group was 45%; the inhibition rate of the nourishing kidney yin experimental group was 44.5%, and the anti-tumor effect of the Buzhong Yiqi experimental group was also 40%. The effect was also good; the tumor inhibition rate of the ATCA mixture experimental group was 36%, and the tumor inhibition rate of the Wenbu Shenyang treatment group was 31%, and the curative effect was poor. It seems that in the suppression of tumors, it is advisable to use a method of tonifying blood and nourishing kidney yin. From the analysis of the survival rate, the qi and blood double supplement group reached 45%, which was the longest survival group; the second was the nourishing kidney yin group, reaching 38.5 ring, the effect was also good, as for the Buzhong Yiqi, Wen The treatment of the kidney-yang and the combination of the ATCA mixture can also prolong the survival period, but it is not as good as the qi and blood supplement and nourishing kidney and yin treatment group. The treatment group of Xiaochaihutang and Fufang Capsules, which are mainly based on cockroaches, showed no significant inhibition of tumors in this group of experiments, and it could not prolong the survival of tumor-bearing mice, and the effect was the worst. Therefore, from the perspective of prolonging the survival period, the treatment of tonifying blood and nourishing kidney and yin is the first choice, followed by Buzhong Yiqi, Wenbu Shenyang and attacking and supplementing. From the two aspects of inhibiting tumor and prolonging survival, the best is to supplement the blood and blood, followed by nourishing kidney yin, followed by Buzhong Yiqi and ATCA mixture. The effect of warming kidney and kidney is not obvious. As for the Xiaochai Hutang and the compound capsules, which are mainly based on cockroaches, there is no obvious effect from the results of this experiment.

In short, each treatment of the righteous and supporting rightness and firming the body-based treatment, both have different degrees of inhibition of tumor growth and prolong survival, while treatment with scorpion venom has no significant inhibition of tumor growth and prolonged survival.

This experiment shows that the treatment of Fuzheng Peiben traditional Chinese medicine or Fuzheng Peiben traditional Chinese medicine is very obvious for tumor suppression of smaller tumors, and can significantly prolong survival and improve quality of life. Therefore, it is often used as one of the auxiliary treatments for postoperative radiotherapy and chemotherapy. Many literatures have reported that the use of Fuzheng Peiben in the treatment of malignant tumors has achieved good results. The results of this experiment further confirm that qi and blood double supplement, nourishing kidney yin, Buzhong Yiqi and other treatments can inhibit tumors and prolong survival. Western medicine combined with clinical treatment of malignant tumors provides experimental basis.

(2)   The role of Fuzheng Peimoto Chinese medicine in enhancing body immunity:

This experiment shows that the traditional Chinese medicine of Fuzheng Pei and the traditional Chinese medicine with Fuzheng Peiben can increase the level of peripheral blood T lymphocytes in different degrees. For example, at the 4th week, the T lymphocyte level is in the Buzhong Yiqi group. %, qi and blood double supplement group 44.8%, nourishing kidney Yin group 38.6%, Wenbu Shenyang group 37.5%, ATCA mixture group 35. 6%; inhibition of thymus atrophy, such as the second week, Buzhong Yiqi The thymus index of the qi and blood double supplement, nourishing kidney yin, warming kidney and aphrodisiac and ATCA mixture treatment group were significantly different from the tumor-bearing control group. It is suggested that the anti-tumor effect of Fuzheng Peiben may be related to enhancing the immune function of the body. Some scholars believe that many plants contain functional components of immunoregulators, called anti-tumor polysaccharides. These polysaccharides cannot directly kill cancer cells, but they can activate the immune system in the body to release cytokines or enhance anti-tumor effects. The killing effect of LAK cells on cancer cells. Fuzheng Pei This medicine is rich in plant polysaccharides. For example, Zhao Kesheng reported that Huangxiao polysaccharide, which has a molecular weight of 20 000-'25 000, is used to secrete tumors in vitro from peripheral blood mononuclear cells (PBMC) of normal people and tumor patients. Necrosis factor (TNF) has a significant promoting effect. Chen Kai et al reported that Chinese herbal compound Fuzheng Kangliu liquid can promote the natural killer cell activity and interleukin-2 (IL-2) activity of transplanted tumor S-180 mice, and It can promote the activation of T lymphocytes, promote the phagocytic function of peritoneal macrophages, and increase the weight of spleen and thymus. In short, the effect of Fuzheng Peiben on the human immune system is very complicated and needs further observation and research.

(3) Fuzheng Peiben Chinese medicine treatment can enhance the body›s disease resistance, enhance blood cells and enhance physical strength:

Experiments have shown that Fuzheng Peimoto can increase the serum protein content of tumor-bearing mice and increase the A/G ratio. The clinical observation data of the author's oncology clinic showed that hepatocarcinoma, esophageal cancer, gastric cancer, and colorectal cancer were treated with xz-C, which is mainly composed of Fuzheng Peiben, and immunoregulatory tumor-inhibiting and removing traditional Chinese medicine. Both red blood cells and hemoglobin were higher than the control group, and leukopenia was also inhibited. It shows that Fuzheng Pei can enhance blood cells and proteins, enhance physical strength and improve disease resistance.

As one of the treatments for the treatment of tumors with integrated Chinese and Western medicine, Fuzheng Peiben has been widely used in clinical practice. The experimental results show that Fuzheng Peiji treatment can delay the time of tumor inoculation, inhibit tumor growth, prolong tumor-bearing survival, enhance immune function and disease resistance, improve quality of life, and can be used for clinical Chinese medicine anticancer research. Provide experimental basis.

3. The immune effect of Chinese herbal medicine on patients with advanced cancer

Patients with advanced cancer are mostly deficient, and common immune function is low. Buxu Fuzheng medicine can enhance the body's immune function and is of great significance for the prevention and treatment of tumor patients with low immune function.

1. Enhance non-specific immune function

(1) It can stimulate the thymus and spleen of the immune organs of animals and increase their weight.
(2) Enhance the phagocytic function of macrophages:
(3) Increase the number of peripheral white blood cells:

2. Enhance cellular immune function

(1)   Promote spleen lymphocyte proliferation:
(2)   Increase the conversion rate of lymphocytes:
(3)   Enhance red blood cell immunity:

3. Enhance humoral immunity

(1)   Promote antibody production:
(2)   Increase the number of spleen antibody forming cells:

8. The New understanding of Cancer Immunotherapy

1. The progress of cancer immunotherapy

Immunotherapy for cancer has been around for nearly a hundred years, and many scholars and clinicians have devoted themselves to the development of this field with great interest in order to make breakthroughs in cancer treatment.

However, after several research booms and peaks, by the 1970s, although cancer immunotherapy had achieved some results in animal experiments and in vitro research,

However, in clinical trials, the results were flat and even disappointing.

Since the 19ᵗʰ century, although the field of immunotherapy has experienced success and failure, scientists have been working hard to explore.

With the further development of immunology research and the accumulation of rich clinical experience, immunotherapy has played an increasingly important role in the treatment of tumors.

Since the 1980s, with the rapid development of cell biology, molecular biology, molecular immunology, genetic engineering and bioengineering technology, it has brought new opportunities and new expectations for cancer immunotherapy.

The introduction of the theory of biological response regulation in 1982 made people re-recognize the theory and practice of traditional immunotherapy, and established the fourth treatment mode for tumors other than surgery, radiotherapy and chemotherapy, namely the biological treatment of tumors.

The establishment of the theory of biological response regulation has provided a theoretical basis for the biological treatment of tumors, and the development and utilization of bioengineering technology has made it possible to clinically apply biological treatment of cancer.

More than 10 cytokines such as interleukin, interferon, tumor necrosis factor, immunoglobulin factor and clone stimulating factor can be produced in large quantities by genetic engineering technology.

Due to the advancement of the above bioengineering technologies and the deep understanding of cellular immunity, molecular immunity, and molecular biology, opportunities for human cancer immunotherapy have been developed.

1) Adoptive immunotherapy, that is, cytotoxic lymphocytes, such as lymphokine-activated killer cells (LAK cells), which have anticancer activity in cancer patients. Clinical studies in patients with advanced cancer have shown that high-dose administration of interleukin-9 alone or in combination with LAK cells can cause tumor regression in some or all of the patients.

2) Injecting patients with IL-2-activated tumor interstitial infiltrating lymphocytes (TIL), which kill cancer cells in animal experiments

The activity is 50-100 times stronger than LAK cells.

3) The combination of various cytokines, such as the combination of interferon or tumor necrosis factor with interleukin-2, and the mass production of recombinant cytokines, can provide a large number of biologically active substances, which may lead to new therapies effective for human cancer. development of.

4) In recent years, some drugs with biological response modifier-like effects have been discovered from traditional Chinese medicine resources, and have achieved gratifying effects in research and clinical applications. These natural drugs with biological response modifier-like effects are undoubtedly a bright future research field by enhancing the body's immune function and activating immune factor activity.

The XZ-C immunomodulatory anticancer Chinese medicine researched by the author is applied to clinical trials based on the success of animal experiments. After 34 years of clinical trials of more than 12, 000 clinical cases, the curative effect is remarkable. XZ-C immunoregulatory Chinese medicine, a natural drug with a biological response regulator-like effect, has achieved gratifying effects in both experimental research and clinical application.

2. Why in the treatment of anti-cancer metastasis must strengthen the immune regulation and control of the host organism

Regarding the important role of strengthening the host immune function against cancer metastasis, **the author has conducted some explorations in animal laboratories and clinical research for more than 60 years.** There are also many reports on the data, according to statistics:

1) The incidence of malignant tumors in patients with primary immunodeficiency is 10,000 times that of the general population of the same age;

2) Organ transplant recipients treated with immunosuppressive drugs, the tumor incidence rate is 100 times that of the general population of the same age;

3) In 135 patients with cancer who have received chemotherapy for a long time, due to suppression of immune function, the number of newly diagnosed malignant lesions has increased greatly;

4) some malignant tumors can be naturally relieved;

5) lymphocytes are not wet in the tumor tissue;

6) he human immune system has the ability to monitor cancer cells.

These examples are sufficient to show that when the body's immune function is low or defective, the body exhibits a low-energy state of immune surveillance for the occurrence and development of tumors. The above phenomenon also provides a basis for immunotherapy to treat tumors.

There are also some data to prove that when the immune function of the body is regulated and restored, it can inhibit the development of tumors. In the 1930s, Willom Coley et al. used "Coley Toxin" to treat patients with advanced tumors. Of the more than 200 patients with various tumors that could be analyzed, more than 30 patients had a survival period of more than 30 years. In the 1980s, Guesada et al. used IFN-a in the treatment of hairy cell leukemia, the effective rate (CR+ PR) was above 90%; in the 1980s, Rosenberg et al treated 228 cases of late metastatic tumor with LAK/IL-2, partial remission 42/228, complete remission 9/228. According to a large amount of data available, immune regulation is one of the important mechanisms for tumorigenesis and development.

3. the body's immune response to tumors and its effect on cancer cells

The immune microenvironment plays an important role in cancer metastasis and recurrence.

It should first be noted that although cancer cells are cells derived from the body's own tissues, they are different from normal cells. The body may use it as a "non-self" cell to produce an antagonistic response, which is a manifestation of the body's immune response. These reactions have been well documented in experimental animals. It is conceivable that in a person's life, a variety of carcinogenic factors cause cell cancer, and are constantly eliminated by the body's immune function and immune cells, and only a few cancerous cells in a few individuals survive, eventually developed into a clinical tumor. Studying the body's immune response to cancer is also of great practical significance in cancer treatment to control the occurrence, development, metastasis and recurrence of cancer.

There have been two different views on the occurrence and development of cancer: one view is that the occurrence and development of a tumor is an "autonomous process" that is basically independent of any defense mechanism of the body. At the treatment of cancer, it rarely pays attention to the regulation of the body's immune system. Another view is that the occurrence and development of **tumors is a "non-autonomous process" or "controlled process" regulated and controlled by various factors in the body, especially immune factors. In view of this point of view, in the treatment policy, we must not only "smash evil spirits", but also pay attention to "righting up".** It is necessary to kill cancer cells, and more attention should be paid to improving the immunity of patients. This will enable more effective control of the development of this process.

In recent years, immunological studies on cancer have shown that the ultimate outcome of cancer metastasis, recurrence, and its evolution depends on the interaction of the biological

properties of the cancer with the body's immune system. Many animal experiments or clinical studies have shown that effective anti-cancer immunity can be stimulated by certain immunomodulation methods. However, cancer can also release immunosuppressive factors to inhibit the body's immune function, reduce host immunity, and evade host immune attacks, to achieve the purpose of escape immune surveillance. <u>**The local micro-environment where the tumor interacts with the body, especially the immune micro-environment, plays an extremely important role in the occurrence, development, metastasis and recurrence of cancer.**</u> A stronger immune microenvironment can effectively control this process, while an immunocompromised immune microenvironment promotes tumorigenesis, development, metastasis, and recurrence.

Clinical studies have found that the true anticancer response in cancer patients is rarely associated with the immune response detected in vitro, suggesting that there are no good assay techniques and data that can accurately reflect the immune function of cancer patients. It is still necessary to further deepen the research to find out the techniques for effectively detecting the immune status of the body and the clinically practical, fast, simple, accurate and effective methods.

Deep research on the changes of **local microenvironment of tumors and the inhibition of tumors on host immune response**, designing immunotherapy programs that target both cancer cells and local microenvironment, effectively stimulate anti-cancer immune function and eliminate micro-cancer It is of great significance to prevent metastasis and recurrence after radical operation.

4. Immune function of cancer patients, especially cellular immune function normally decreases with tumor development

Cancer patients can escape immune attack by passive escaping way and active suppression of host immune function, which are two ways to evade the host immune attack.

Some studies about cancer localized immune status show that immune cells infiltrating cancerous tissues is greater than in the cancer tissue infiltration of immune cells, suggesting that within the cancerous tissue infiltration of immunocompetent cells is low. This result suggests that, although within the cancerous tissue infiltration of immune cells is low, there may be tumor-bearing host immune system deficiencies, but still have normal T cell response. In animal experiments and clinical studies an effective anti-tumor immunity can be stimulated, which the key is how to break the cancer suppression for the immune system, stimulate effective immune response, especially in T cell-based immune response.

The inferior immunologic functions of carcinoma patients, especially the abnormal local immunologic micro-environment of the tumor, resulting in ineffective immune defence reaction of the body, is the important factor for the carcinoma to meet with immunologic escape and metastasis and reoccurrence easily. How to effectively regulate the immunologic functions of the host, how to improve the local micro-environment of the tumor so as to be good to bring the anti-carcinoma effect of the host into play and how to improve the micro-environment obstacle to reduce the implantation of the metastatic lesion of the cancer cells are the important and effective measures to prevent the reoccurrence and metastasis of carcinoma after operation, eliminate the metastatic lesion due to the implantation of the remained cancer cells in the chest cavity and abdominal cavity after operation

5. tumor immunosuppression

1). *The occurrence, development and metastasis, recurrence are closely related to hypoplasia of the immune system and decrease immune function in cancer*
   (1)   The body's immune system dysfunction and decreased immune function are prone to cancer:

An animal neonatal had thymectomy; chemotherapy drugs, radiation and adrenal hormones, etc. can inhibit the body's immune status so that the virus induces cancer and tumors xenograft successfully. In addition, the patients with the acquired immunodeficiency, and long-term use of immunosuppressive drugs or long-term use of chemotherapy patients have higher incidence of cancer.

   (2)   Malignant tumor directly violates immune organs and causes immune dysfunction or inhibition and also releases immunosuppressive factors which reduce host immune or induces to increase suppressor cells in vivo. Clinically, patients with advanced malignancies generally had low immune function, but after surgery removed the tumor and the situation of the diseases was remissed, immune function had different degrees of recovery.

2). *The performance of tumor immune suppression can show as the following four aspects*
   (1)   Suppressor Cells: are mostly suppressor T cells (TS cells) and inhibiting macrophage.

Tumor-bearing mice TS cells cultured in vitro can be released specifically inhibit factor, directly on the effector cells, inhibit the cytotoxic effect of CTL. For some tumors from immunosuppressive macrophages, peripheral blood mononuclear cells inhibit LAK cell activity. The results showed that the tumor cells and macrophages PEG: or some humoral factors, can inhibit LAK cells.

   (2)   Producing abnormal lymphokines:

In tumor progression, not only in tumor-bearing cell host immune function abnormalities, and lymphokines function also disorders such as IFN-y and IL-2, etc., studies confirm that tumor growth and progression of IFN-y and IL-2 production generating a negative correlation, it is suggested that lymphokine tumor-bearing host an exception has become an important cause of tumor immune escape.

(3)　immunosuppressive cytokine production

①tumor-derived immune suppressor.
From the discovery of one mouse fibrosarcoma tumor-derived inhibitory factor (tumor derived suppressor factor, TDSF) can induce TS cells. Some tumor cells can secrete prostaglandins (PEG2), transforming growth factor-p (TGF- groups, and other load-inhibiting substance; hepatocellular carcinoma can secrete AFP, these substances are immunosuppressive and its reaction more effector cell function was inhibited, such as LAK cells, lymphocytes, macrophages.

② soluble interleukin-2 receptor .IL-2 receptor (IL-2R) expression in activated T cells, NK cells, macrophages cell membrane still bound to the surface, IL-2R down and become free of soluble interleukin-2 receptor (sIL-2R) after IL-2, may also reduce the activity of IL-2 .SIL-2R is a soluble T cell activation markers substance, T cells, B cells, macrophages, and lymphokine-activated killer cells could express SJL-2R0 SIL-2R also inhibit IL-2 stimulation of peripheral lymphocytes killing live · wins.

(4)　Abnormal function of the effective cells

A.NK cells
in the human and mouse lymphocytes in a class of killer cells, both without stimulation by antigen and does not require participation of the antibody, so called natural killer cells in patients with tumor suppressor T cells, inhibiting single nucleated cells, suppressor macrophages produce PEG2, while tumor cells also produce PEG2 .PEG: inhibit NK activity of NK cell activity and therefore the majority of cancer patients are relatively low

B.LAK cells namely lymphokine activated killer. cells, its most prominent feature is a broad-spectrum anti-tumor effect.

LAK precursor cells mainly by NK cells and T cells. LAK cells in the peripheral blood NK cells come from. Macrophages and inhibit the immunosuppressive cytokine production, can inhibit the activity of LAK cells. Therefore, with the growth of tumors, peripheral blood LAK cell activity tends to decrease.

6. the immune escape of cancer cells

Immune surveillance plays a key role in the development of the immune system in identifying and interfering with malignant tumors. <u>Immune surveillance was originally proposed by F. M. Burnet. He believes that the thymus-dependent immune cells, T lymphocytes, constantly scan the body for abnormal changes and destroy the damaged cells.</u>

The immune escape of cancer cells refers to the immune surveillance of cancer cells that escape the host and keep the cancer cells from attack by the host and continue to grow. This involves the biological characteristics of cancer cells, the immune status of the body, and the potential between the two. There are a series of immune surveillance mechanisms in the body, but cancer cells may still evade the body's immune attack and immune surveillance through a variety of mechanisms.

1). The antigenicity of cancer cells is weak or the antigen is reduced.

Most tumor cells are weakly immunogenic and do not elicit a potent anti-tumor immune response, or the host's immune response to tumor antigens results in a reduction or loss of tumor cell surface antigens, such that tumor cells are not recognized by the immune system.

2). Tissue-compatible complex (MHC) expression is abnormal.

The expression of MHC class 1 antigen on the surface of some tumor cells is reduced or absent, so that the CTL does not recognize the antigen on the tumor cells, so that the tumor cells can escape the host's immune attack.

3). The surface of the tumor cells is "antigen capped" or blocked.

Tumor cell surface antigens may be covered by certain substances. For example, tumor cells can express high levels of salivary glycopolysaccharide or a tumor-activated agglutination system, both of which can cover tumor antigens and thus cannot be host lymphocytes. Identification, it will not play a killing effect. The presence of a blocking factor in the serum blocks the antigenic determinants on the surface of the tumor cells, thereby allowing the cancer cells to escape the recognition of the effector cells and the immune-sensing lymphocytes to attack.

4). The down-regulation of tumor cell antigen processing cannot present specific antigens to host T cells, which may be one of its immune immune monitoring mechanisms.
5). Adhesion molecule is a kind of membrane surface glycoprotein that mediates the adhesion between cells and extracellular matrix (ECM), and plays an important role in tumor progression and metastasis. It also plays a role in tumor escape immune attack, such as abnormal expression of certain Weng's molecules, which can make tumor cells escape the immune surveillance of T cells.

Immunogenic tumor cells are easily destroyed by the body.

Spontaneous tumors with very weak antigenicity cannot induce an effective anti-tumor immune response, thus evading immune surveillance and selective survival and proliferation. Because the amount of early tumor cells is small, it is not enough to stimulate the body's immune system to produce sufficient immune response, and when the tumor grows to a certain extent, a tumor cell group is formed. At this time, the tumor antigen coding gene has been mutated, which may interfere with the immune recognition process. Tumor cells are leaking. **This phenomenon is called sneakin through of tumor cells or** tumor cells escape (sneakin through),

During tumor formation, certain tumors that are sensitive to immune surveillance are eliminated, and insensitive tumors survive. This phenomenon is called "immunoselection", the decline or antigenicity of tumor antigens during tumor growth. Very weak spontaneous tumors do not induce an effective anti-tumor immune response, or are insensitive to immune smear, thus evading the body's immune surveillance and selective survival and proliferation.

7. The important role in cancer immunotherapy during anti-cancer metastasis

Cancer is indeed one of the most serious diseases, and various existing conventional treatment methods are also grim. Surgery and radiation therapy for cancer are not specific. Surgery for cancer is completely non-selective, and radiation therapy is generally more effective for rapidly dividing cells. whether surgical or radiotherapy is local treatment, which solves only the problem of localized cancer without systemic therapeutic effect. Surgery kills cancer cells by Zero-order kinetics which means that all being treated cells (tumor resection) were killed. On the other hand, radiation therapy is a kinetic (first-order Kinetics), that is each treatment kills only a certain percentage of the treated cells. Therefore, radiation treatment cannot be completely eliminated tumor cell mass that cannot kill the last remaining cell.

Chemotherapy is fairly reasonable toxic pharmaceutically. The toxic effects of these drugs are due to non-specific, non-selective, not only kill cancer cells but also kill normal cells. Radiation therapy with these drugs are the same as radiation therapy which is first-order kinetics and often cannot be completely eliminated tumor, but its role is systemic, and therefore it has effect on disseminated disease. Moreover, surgery, radiotherapy and chemotherapy decrease immunity of the host; radiotherapy and chemotherapy also suppress bone marrow function; cytotoxic chemotherapy has impairment on the liver and renal function and has severe toxicity, in which patients suffer deeply.

However, in theory immunotherapy should be the best treatment. Because:

(1) It has a sensitive specific immunologically, it only affects the cancer cells without harming normal cells all. So it is non-toxic and non-invasive treatment (radiotherapy and chemotherapy was toxic and damaging treatment).

(2) its role is systemic, it can be used in the treatment of disseminated disease.

(3) If the cancer antigen by immunization with special effects, it should be subject to all of the tumor cells genus 0 kinetics role.

(4) no deformity, no dysfunction.

Immunotherapy works differently than chemotherapy and rarely eliminates large tumors. In animal model studies as well as in human studies, immunotherapy is effective for those with small tumors or a small number of residual lesions (subclinical lesions or tumors that are not visible to the naked eye). Immunotherapy is most suitable for treating cancer cells that are undergoing metastasis. The future role of immunotherapy may be as a combination of other "reduced cell" treatments, such as surgery, radiotherapy and chemotherapy, which these therapies are effective in reducing cancer cells in patients, but often do not completely eliminate the lesions. Some scholars believe that immunotherapy can be used as an auxiliary treatment for surgery.

<u>Whether adjuvant therapy is needed after surgical resection of primary malignant tumors has become a problem that must be considered in cancer treatment</u>. In the past, it was believed that regional lymph nodes were an effective barrier to systemic dissemination of tumors, thus emphasizing local and regional treatment of primary tumors.

Although modern surgical and radiotherapy techniques have significantly reduced primary and regional tumor recurrence rates, there has been no significant change in survival rates for all patients over the past 30 years. <u>This fact highlights the need for a systemic approach</u>.

It is now clear that regardless of the tissue type or anatomy of a malignant tumor, as long as regional lymph node metastasis is present, 70% -80% of treatment failures are predicted. Therefore, rather than the regional lymph node is a barrier to the spread of lesions, it is better to say that it indicates a high probability of distant metastasis. Because the regional lymph node is an intermediate station, it will eventually enter the blood circulation through the thoracic duct. Thus, regional lymph node positive should be considered as a staging index, suggesting that the treatment should exceed the range of the primary tumor and its regional lymphoid tissue.

At present, the effective treatment for systemic therapy, that is, the treatment of cancer cells during metastasis, is only chemotherapy and immunotherapy, biological therapy, Chinese medicine treatment, and combination of Chinese and Western medicine. Physicians must consider a new set of treatment options when considering asymptomatic patients, clinically non-metastatic, but potentially active lesions. This ideal adjuvant anticancer regimen must act on the body, be specific to cancer cells and relatively non-toxic. These two effective effects on systemic treatment---chemotherapy and immunotherapy, the specificity of immunotherapy for cancer cells has shown a good development prospect. Therefore, great attention and energy have been given to both its foundation and clinical practice. Some of the principles derived from tumor immunology are beneficial, such as the following clinical studies.

(1)   lung cancer;

Amery et al. compared a group of lung cancer patients who underwent surgical resection with surgical resection plus postoperative L-wine treatment in a European collaborative trial group. 178 patients have been observed so far, and the trend of better efficacy in patients receiving adjuvant levofloxacin is seen. Takita et al reported a group of very advanced but resectable stage n lung cancers and received adjuvant immunotherapy. Treatment of 6. Most of the patients achieved initial results. Although preliminary, these reports seem to indicate that postoperative adjuvant immunotherapy is effective in patients with lung cancer.

(2)   Colon cancer:

Ongoing colon cancer-assisted immunotherapy appears to have no improvement in the latter than the effect of chemotherapy with only fluorourethane and chemotherapy plus BCG.

(3)   Breast cancer:

Spark et al. compared the chemotherapy of stage II breast cancer with chemical immunotherapy. The preliminary results indicate that chemical immunotherapy has obvious effects on patients.

8. How to Evaluate Immunity Measure, BRM Treatment and Curative Effect and Value of Chinese Traditional Medicines Similar to BRM

As to the evaluation standard of the curative effect, there are two different understandings.

The traditional curative measure holds that the evaluation standard of the curative effect is: the traditional therapeutics concept of the carcinoma holds that the cancerous protuberance is caused by the crazy cleavage and proliferation of the cells, so the cancer cells are the arch criminal. Therefore, the target of tackling the key problem is to kill off the cancer cells and the therapeutic methods include operation, radiotherapy and chemotherapy and the objective or target of the treatment is the primary lesion or (and) metastatic lesion. The evaluation standard of the curative effects of the three largest traditional treatment measures is to relieve the primary carcinoma block or the shrinkage or disappear of the metastatic lesion, in other words, it takes the tumor as the evaluation standard.

XU ZE New Concept holds: the goal of tackling the key problem is the metastasis. **It is necessary to pay attention to the treatment of the primary lesion and metastatic lesion as well as the treatment of the cancer cells in routing of metastasis. These cancer cells or cancer cell groups or micro- thrombus in the routing of metastasis cannot be seen or touched at present or be displayed through iconography such as B ultrasonic, CT and MRI and so on, therefore, it cannot evaluate it through the size of the carcinoma lesion.** Generally, the evaluation standard for the curative effect of the chemotherapy is relief and shrinkage. However, relief and shrinkage are not the goal of treatment of the carcinoma patient, "being effective" that it means only refers to the shrinkage of the cancerous protuberance and it does not obviously prolong the life of the carcinoma patient and improve the survival quality of the patient. The basis to evaluate the shrinkage is generally the size of the occupation of the iconography such as B ultrasonic, CT and X-ray, which is very scientific, correct and reasonable. Shrinkage is better than non-shrinkage. However, it is not so absolute. Some cancerous protuberances shrink, but they meet with metastasis rapidly; some do not meet with shrinkage or metastasis. Maybe the occupation is small, but inside it are the cancer cells; or the occupation lesion may be large, there are not only the cancer cells but also the liquefacient organization with cellular necrosis inside it. In the recent 34 years, we have seen from so many metastatic and recurrent patients from time to time in Shuguang Tumor Clinic that the tumor is obviously shrunk after radiotherapy and chemotherapy, however, the patients meet with reoccurrence and metastasis after a long time or several months; after radiotherapy, there is a little metastasis; after chemotherapy, it is easy to meet with metastasis. In this tumor clinic, after assistant chemotherapy, ***it was found by us that some patients met with fewer metastasis when they were subject to chemotherapy not exceeding 4 times after operation compared to the ones subject to over 4 chemotherapies***. The more the chemotherapy times, the easier the remote metastasis, chemotherapy while metastasis, more chemotherapy, more metastasis. Maybe the radiotherapy is the local treatment and the chemotherapy acts on the whole body, killing off the cancer cells in the whole body as well as the immunological cells and stem cells in the whole body, making the whole immunologic function inferior, making the immunological survelillance of the body of the host weakened, in this way, the remote metastasis may easily appear, it even promotes the metastasis. With respect to the evaluation of its curative effect and value, the more important is to whether it prevents the occurrence of the metastatic lesion and controls the metastasis. Since one of the goal of carcinoma treatment is to improve the immunity of the patient and improve the inhibition ability of the host to the carcinoma. Anti metastasis is to control the cancer cells in routing of metastasis and improve the immunological surveillance of the blood circulation system. The immunity treatmemt or BRM treatmemt or Z-C immune regulation medicine similar to **BRM that can kill off 10^5~10^6** cancer cells, cannot make the primary lesion or metastatic lesion shrink or disappear, however, the new metastatic lesions obviously reduces or no new metastatic lesions appear any more, controlling the metastasis. Therefore, if the immunity treatment is evaluated with the shrinkage of the carcinoma lesion, its curative effect is just so so. If it improves the survival quality and prolongs the survival period through improve the immunological surveillance of the body of the host and kill off or inhibit the cancer cells in routing of metastasis, its effect is very remarkable. Immunity measure and the therapy with Z-C immune regulation and anti-tumor medicine can obviously improve the survival quality of the patients, improve the symptom, enhance the body condition, improve the spirit and appetite for food, obviously prolong the survival period and improve the long-term curative effect.

9. Experimental Study and Observation of Its Clinical Curative Effects on Treatment of Malignant Tumore with XZ-C Traditional Chinese Anti-cancer Immunologic Regulation and Control Medication

In order to look for the traditional herb medicine with actually curative effect and without toxication and adverse reaction, this surgical tumor research institute has screened 200 kinds of Chinese herbal medicines with so-called anticancer reaction recorded on Chinese herbal medicine books for tumor-inhibition reaction on the solid carcinoma in the tumor-bearing animal models one by one in the past 4 years. Through long-term in-vivo tumor-inhibiting animal experiments, we have screened 48 kinds of Chinese herbal medicines with relatively good tumor-inhibition rate that can prolong the survival time, protect the immune organ and obviously improve the immunologic function. According to the clinical conditions, the anticancer medicines screened are combined into 2 compounds including $Z-C_1$ and $Z-C_4$ with better anti-cancer reaction than each single medicine. In the original screening, we carried out the tumor-inhibiting animal experiment for each single medicine and now we further carry out the experimental study on these two groups of compounds for the tumor-inhibiting reaction in the solid tumor of the tumor-bearing rats.

1. Experimental Study on Animal

1). Materials and Method

(1) Experimental animal: 260 Kunming clon white rats, half of male and female respectively, weight:21±2g, 8~10 weeks.

(2) Cell strains and inoculation: hepatic carcinoma H_{22} cell strains, the fresh tumor bodies from the rats with tumor were prepared into the single cell suspended liquid, after dyeing and counting of the cancer cells (1×10^6/ml), 0.2ml normal saline of cancer cell was subject to subcutaneous vaccination at the front axilla at the right side of each rat.

(3) Drugs and experimental group: the traditional herb medicines $Z-C_1$ and $Z-C_4$ were entirely developed and prepared by Hubei Branch of China Anti-cancer Research Cooperation of Chinese Traditional Medicine and Western Medicine, the former was a compound and the latter was a medicinal powder. The chemotherapy control medicine used by the chemotherapy group was cyclophosphane (CTX).

Experimental group: the animals with H_{22} cancer cell transplanted were divided into four groups randomly: ① traditional herb medicine $Z-C_1$ group (90 rats). The rats were subject to gastriclavage once every day after 24h of transplantation of cancer cells, 0.8ml per rat every time, equivalent to 1.4mg of the dried medicinal herbs. ②Traditional herb medicine $Z-C_4$ group (90 rats), as to the dose and gastriclavage method, ditto. ③Chemotherapy group (50 rats), from the next day after transplantation of cancer cells, they were subject to gastriclavage with CTX50mg/kg weight every other day. ④Control group (30 rats), they were subject to gastriclavage with normal saline every day from the next day after transplantation of the cancer cells, 0.8ml/rat.

(4) Observation of indexes: measure the weight of the rats every 3d, measure the diameter of the tumor with vernier caliper, measure the immunologic function and blood picture. Half of each group as Group A, subject to tumor-bearing experiment, regular killing of the rats in batches, separation of tumor and weighing of the tumor and then calculation of tumor-inhabiting rate. The tumor was subject to the pathological section and a few of the specimens were subject to the observation of ultra-structural organization. The rest half of each group as Group B. The tumor-bearing experimental rats were drenched for a long time until they met with natural death. Then the tumor was separated and weighed, the long-term inhibition rate and life elongation rate of the tumor was calculated.

2). Experimental result

(1) The tumor-inhibition effect of Z-C Medicine on Rats bearing hepatic carcinoma H_{22}: in the second week after administration of $Z-C_1$, the tumor-inhibition rate was 40% and the one in the fourth week was 45% and 58% in the sixth week. The tumor-inhibition rate after administration of $Z-C_4$ was 55%, 68% in the fourth week and 70% in the sixth week. (P<0.01) the tumor-inhibiting rate after administration of CTX was 45% in the second week, 45% in the fourth week and 49% in the sixth week (See Fig.1 and 2).

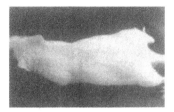 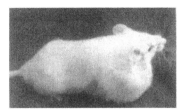

Fig. 1 Z-C$_1$ and Z-C$_4$ therapy group   Fig. 2 Control group

30d after inoculation of hepatic   30d after inoculation of hepatic
carcinoma H$_{22}$ carcinoma H$_{22}$

(2) The effect of Z-C medicine on the survival time of the rats bearing hepatic carcinoma H$_{22}$: the average survival time of Z-C$_1$, Z-C$_4$ and CTX was longer than the one of the normal saline control group (P<0.01); Z-C medicine played a role in obviously prolonging the survival time. Through comparison with the control group, the life elongation rate of Z-C$_1$ group was 85%, the one of Z-C$_4$ group was 200% and the one of CTX group was 9.8%. The rats in Z-C$_1$ and CTX in Group B met with death in 75d. 6 rats bearing carcinoma in Z-C$_4$ survived after seven months.

(3) Both Z-C$_1$ and Z-C$_4$ medicine improved the immunologic function and Z-C$_4$ obviously improved the immunologic function, increased the white blood cells and red blood cells, without any effect on the hepatic function and kidney function and without damage to the hepatic and kidney section. CTX decreased the white blood cells and reduced the immunologic function with the renal damage to the kidney section. The thymus in the control group was obviously atrophic (Fig. 1-4) while the one of Z-C$_1$ and Z-C$_2$ therapy group was not atrophic but a little hypertrophic (Fig.1-3).

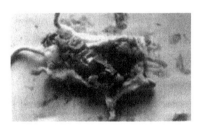 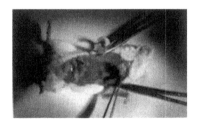

Fig. 3 Z-C$_4$ therapy group   Fig. 4 Control group

The thymus was obviously hypertrophic   The thymus was obviously atrophic
in 30 days after inoculation of hepatic   in 30 days after inoculation of
carcinoma H$_{22}$ hepatic carcinoma H$_{22}$

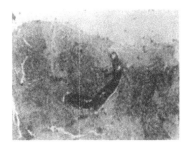

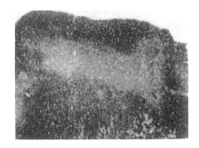

Fig. 5 Pathological section of the thymus in tumor-bearing control group

HE x 100 cortex atrophia lymphocyte

Fig. -6 Thymus of Z-C4 control group

HE x 100 the cortex and medulla of the thymus built up and the lymphocyte was highly dense

Pathological section of thymus in the control group: the cortex of the thymus was atrophic, the cells were discrete and the blood vessel met with sludge (Fig. 1-5). The pathological section of the thymus in Z-C$_4$ therapy group displayed that the cortical area of the thymus built up, the lymphocyte was dense, the epithelium reticulocyte increased and the thymus corpuscles increased (Fig. 1-6).

2. Observation on Clinic Application

1. Clinical information

(1) Hubei Branch of China Anti-cancer Research Cooperation of Chinese Traditional Medicine and Western Medicine, Anti Carcinoma Metastasis and Recurrence Research Office and Shuguang Tumor Specialized Outpatient Department had treated 4, 698 carcinoma patients in Stage III and IV or in metastasis and recurrence with Z-C medicine combined with western medicine from 1994 to Nov. 2002, among which there were 3, 051 men patients and 1,647 women patients. The youngest one was 11 years old and the oldest one was 86 years old, the high invasion age was 40~69 years. All groups of the patients were entirely subject to the diagnosis of pathological histology or definitive diagnosis with ultrasonic B, CT and MRI iconography. According to the staging standard of UICC, all the cases were entirely the patients in medium and advanced stage over Stage III. In this group, there were 1,021 hepatic carcinoma patients, among which there were 694 primary lesion hepatic carcinoma patients and 327 metastatic hepatic carcinoma patients; there were 752 patients suffering from carcinoma of lung, among which there were 699 patients suffering from the primary carcinoma of lung and 53 patients suffering from the metastatic carcinoma of lung; there were 668 gastric carcinoma patients, 624 patients suffering from esophagus cardia carcinoma, 328 patients suffering from rectum carcinoma of anal canal, 442 patients suffering from carcinoma of colon, 368 patients suffering from breast carcinoma, 74 patients

suffering from adenocarcinoma of pancreas, 30 patients suffering from carcinoma of bile duct, 43 patients suffering from retroperitoneal tumor, 38 patients suffering from oophoroma, 9 patients suffering from cervical carcinoma, 11 patients suffering from cerebroma, 34 patients suffering from thyroid carcinoma, 38 patients suffering from nasopharyngeal carcinoma, 9 patients suffering from melanoma, 27 patients suffering from kidney carcinoma, 48 patients suffering from carcinoma of urinary bladder, 13 patients suffering from leukemia, 47 patients suffering from metastasis of supraclavicular lymph nodes, 35 patients suffering various fleshy tumors and 39 patients suffering from other malignancies.

(2) Medicine and medication: the treatment aims to support healthy energy to eliminate evils, soften and resolve the hard mass and supplement qi and blood. $Z-C_1$ is the compound, 150ml to be taken on the daily basis, $Z-C_4$ is powder, 10g to be taken on the daily basis. According to the analysis and differentiation of the diseases, anti-cancer powder shall be taken orally and the anti-cancer apocatastasis paste shall be applied externally for the solid tumor or the metastatic tumor. In case of being in pain, anti-cancer aponic paste shall be applied externally. Icterus removal soup or dropsy removal soup shall be taken orally for the patients suffering from icterrus and the ascites.

(3) Therapeutic evaluation: it pays attention to the short-term curative effect and iconography indexes as well as the survival time of long-term curative effect, quality of life and immunologic indexes. Attention shall be paid to the changes in subjective signs in administration of drugs. It will be effective when the subjective signs are improved and last over one month; otherwise, it will be ineffective. As to the quality of life (Karnofsky Performance Status), it will be effective when it is improved and lasts over one month, otherwise, it will be ineffective. As to the evaluation standard of the curative effect of solid tumor, it can be divided into four levels according to the changes in size of tumor: Level I: disappearance of tumor; Level II: tumor reduces 1/2; Level III: softening of tumor; Level IV: no change or enlargement of level tumor.

2. Curative results

(1) The symptom was improved, the quality of life was improved, the survival time was prolonged: among the 4,277 carcinoma patients in medium and advanced stage who took Z-C medicine with the return visit over 3 months, the case history had the specific observation record of the curative effect, see Table 1-1. It improved the quality of life of the patients in an all-round way, see Table 1-2.

Table 1-1 General information about 4,277 patients suffering from recurrence and metastasis

		Hepatic carcinoma	Carcinoma of lung	Gastric carcinoma	Esophagus cardia carcinoma	Rectum carcinoma of anal canal	Carcinoma of colon	Breast carcinoma	adenocarcinoma of pancreas
No. of cases		1 021	752	668	624	328	442	368	74
Male: female		4:1	4.4:1	2.25:1	3.1:1	1:1	2.1:1	Female	3.2:1
Focus	Primary	694 (68.6%)	699 (93.9%)						
	Metastasis	327 (31.2%)	53 (6.1%)						
Usual metastasis part in this group		Metastatic lung (2) From the stomach (31.2%)	Metastasis of supraclavicular lymph nodes (11.6%)	Metastatic lever (23.8%) Lung metastasis (3%)	Upper metastasis of compact bone (13.1%)	Reoccurrence rate (14.8%)	Metastatic lever (16.0%)	Metastasis of supraclavicular lymph nodes (17.5%)	Metastatic lever (11.7%)
		From esophagus cardia (19.5%) From recta (31.2%)	Brain metastasis (3.1%) Bone metastasis (4.6%)	Metastasis of peritoneum (29.1%) Upper metastasis of compact bone (6.1%)	Metastatic lever (8.3%)	Metastatic lever (7.0%)	Metastasis of peritoneum (6.0%)	Metastasis of axillary lymph nodes (15.0%) Bone metastasis (5.0%)	Rear metastasis of peritoneum (39.1%)
Age	high invasion (year) %	30~39 (76.2)	50~69 (71.6)	40~49 (73.4)	40~69 (80.4)	40~49 (75.2)	30~69 (88.0)	40~59 (65.9)	40~59 (70.0)
	Oldest (year) %	11	20	17	30	27	27	29	34
	Youngest (year) %	86	80	77	77	78	76	80	68

Table 1-2 Observation of curative effect on 4 277 patients: fully improving the quality of life of the carcinoma patients in medium and advanced stage

Improvement	Vigor	Appetite	Reinforcement of physical force	Improvement in generalized case	Increase of body weight	Improvement of sleep	The restriction of improvement activity and capability released activity	self servicing normal walking	Resumption of work Engaged in light work
No. of cases (%)	4071	3986	2450	479	2938	1005	1038	3220	479
	95.2	93.2	57.3	11.2	68.7	23.5	24.3	75.3	11.2

In this group, all of them were the patients in medium and advanced stage. After taking the medicine, their symptoms were improved to different extents with the effective rate of 93.2%. With respect to the improvement of the quality of life (as per Karnofsky Performance Status), it rose to 80 scores on average after administration from 50 on average before administration; the patients in this group met with the different metastasis and dysfunction of the organs about Stage III. It was reported by the previous statistic information that the mesoposition survival time of this kind of patients was about 6 months. The longest time among this group of the cases reached up to 11 years; another patient suffering from hepatic carcinoma had taken Z-C medicine for ten years and a half; two patients suffering from hepatic carcinoma met with frequency encountered carcinomatous lesion in the left and right liver and it entirely subsided through secondary CT reexamination after the patient took Z-C medicine for half a year and the state of the disease had been stable over half a year. One patient suffering from double-kidney carcinoma met with the widespread metastasis of abdominal cavity after removal of one kidney, after taking Z-C medicine, he was entirely recovered and began to work again. 3 patients suffering from carcinoma of lung, with the lung not removed through explaraton, had taken Z-C medicine over three years and a half. 2 patients suffering from gastric remnant carcinoma had taken Z-C medicine for 8 years. 3 patients suffering from reoccurrence of rectal carcinoma had taken Z-C medicine for 3 years. 1 patient suffering from metastatic liver and rib of the mastocarcinoma had taken Z-C medicine for 8 years. 1 patient suffering from the recurrent bladder carcinoma after operation of renal carcinoma had not met with the carcinoma for 9 years and a half after taking Z-C medicine. All of these patients were the ones in the medium and advanced stage that could not be operated once more or treated with radiotherapy or chemotherapy. They only took Z-C medicine without other medicines for treatment. Up to today, they are reexamined and get the medicine at the out-patient department every month. Through taking the medicine for a long time, the state of the disease is controlled in the stable state to make the organism and the tumor in balanced state for a relatively long time and get a relatively good survival with tumor, in this way, the symptoms of the patients are improved, the quality of life is improved and the survival time is prolonged.

(2) As to 84 patients suffering from solid tumor and 56 patients suffering from enlargement of upper lymph node of metastatic compact bone, after taking Z-C series medicines orally and applying Z-C3 anti-cancer apocatastasis paste, they met with good curative effects, see table 1-3.

Table 1-3 Changes of 84 patients suffering from solid tumor and 56 patients suffering from metastatic mode after applying Z-C paste externally

	Solid tumor				Enlargement of upper lymph node of metastatic compact bone			
	Disappearance	Shrinkage 1/2	Softening	No change	Disappearance	Shrinkage 1/2	Softening	No change
No. of cases (%)	12	28	32	12	12	22	14	8
	14.2	33.3	38.0	14.2	21.4	39.2	25.0	14.2
Total effective rate (%)		85.7				85.7		

115

(3) 298 patients suffering from carcinoma pain obtained the obvious pain alleviation effects after taking Z-C medicine orally and applying Z-C anti-cancer apocatastasis paste externally, see Table 1-4.

Clinical menifetation	Pain		Disappearance	Avoidance
	Light alleviation	Obvious alleviation		
No of cases	52	139	93	14
(%)	17.3	46.8	31.2	4.7
Total effective rate (%)	95.3			

3. Discussion about Z-C Medicine Experiment and Clinic Curative Effect

1). Tumor-inhibition effect of Z-C$_{1-4}$ Medicine on hepatic carcinoma H$_{22}$ rats bearing tumor

It was found that after the medicine was taken to H$_{22}$ tumor-bearing rats for two weeks, four weeks and six weeks, the tumor inhibition rate increased with the prolongation of the administration time, the tumor inhibition rate of Z-C$_4$ in the 6th week reached up to 70%. Through two repeated experiments in succession, the results were stable, which indicated that the tumor-inhibition effect of Chinese herb medicine was slow and it would increase gradually, that is to say, the tumor-inhibition effect was of positive correlation to the accumulated dosage of Chinese herb medicine.

The effect on the survival time of hepatic carcinoma H$_{22}$ tumor-bearing rats from Z-C$_1$ and Z-C$_4$ medicine: it was proven by the experimental results that Z-C$_1$ and Z-C$_4$ medicine could obviously prolong the survival time of the tumor-bearing rats, especially Z-C$_4$, it could prolong the survival time as long as 200%, more than that, Z-C$_4$ could remarkably improve the immunologic function of the organism, protect the immune organ and the bone marrow, alleviate the toxic action and side effect of the radiotherapy and chemotherapy medicines. Furthermore, no toxic action or side effect had been found in the past 12 months after the rats took the medicine. The above-mentioned experimental study offered the beneficial basis to the clinical application.

2). Clinical curative effect

Based on the experimental study, it had been applied to various clinical carcinomas, most of the patients were the ones over Stage III and IV, namely: the ones suffering from the cancer of late stage that could not be removed with exploratory operation; the ones with the exploratory operation without operation indication; the ones meeting with metastasis or reoccurrence in short term or long term after operation of the carcinoma; the ones suffering from hepatic metastasis, lung metastasis or brain metastasis or with cancerous pleural effusion or cancerous ascites in late stage; the ones suffering from various carcinomas conservative removal operation with the exploratory operation only for the anastomosis of intestines and stomach or colostomy but not for removal and the ones not suitable for the operation, chemotherapy and radiotherapy and so on. Through over 10 years' clinical application and systematic observation, $Z-C_1$ and $Z-C_4$ medicine had obtained remarkable curative effect and no toxic action and side effect had been found after long-term administration. It had been proven by the clinical observation that $Z-C_1$ and $Z-C_4$ medicine could improve the survival quality of the carcinoma patients in medium and late stage in an all-round way, improve the whole immunity, control the hyperplasia of the cancer cells, consolidate and enhance the long-term curative effect. The oral-taken and external-applied Z-C medicine had good curative effect in softening and shrinking body surface metastatic tumor. With the assistance of intervention or treatment with cannula spray pump for medicine, it could protect liver, kidney and bone marrow hemopoietic system and the immune organ and improve the immune function.

3). Good pain alleviation effect of Z-C anti-cancer pain alleviation paste

Pain is the relatively remarkable and painful symptom of the carcinoma patients in late stage, the common pain reliever had no remarkable effect on carcinoma pain, the stupefacient pain reliever had the addiction and dependence, Z-C anti-cancer pain alleviation paste had strong pain alleviation effect with a long maintenance time. It was proven through 298 cases of clinical verification that the effective rate was 78.0%, the total effective rate was 95.3%, after repeated application, there were no toxic action or side effect, without addiction. The paid alleviation effect was stable and it was an effective therapeutic method for the carcinoma patients to get rid of the pain and improve the quality of life.

Through experimental research and clinical validation, our experience is: Chinese medicine with Chinese characteristics has its unique advantage in cancer treatment, such as a strong overall concept, conditioning prominent role, mild side effects, can relieve pain, relieve symptoms, and significantly improved quality of life of patients, can mobilize the body's immune function and overall disease resistance, improve the therapeutic effect.

4. The research on cytokine induction factors of XZ-C anticancer immune regulation and control medication

1). $XZ-C_4$ induces endogenous cytokines

(1) Through the experiments: $XZ-C_4$ has many immune strengthening functions and has closely relationship to the induced endogenous cytokines
(2) $XZ-C_4$ can recover the reduction of the white blood cells, granulation cells and platelets.
(3) $XZ-C_4$ can have the direct function on GM-CSF production from granulation cell (GM) through IL-1 β, also increase TNF, IFN etc all of kind of the cell factors, which are possible the indirect function.

(4) $XZ-C_4$ can increase the Th1 cell factors, which were decrease in the cancer patients. There are the curative effects on the anemia and the white blood cells decrease due to the chemotherapy.

(5) The experiment analysis showed that $XZ-C_4$ not only protects the bone marrow function, but also has direct function on the tumor cell division.

In brief, $XZ-C_4$ can induce the tumor division and natural death through the autocrine which produce all of kind of factors. The autocrine is the secretory things from the host to affect the host's function. $XZ-C_4$ probably will become the induction therapy to the tumor division in the future.

2). $XZ-C_4$ inhibiting cancer development and metastasis

The malignant development is defined as tumor cells accepting invasion and metastasis characters during the proliferation. Cancer research need to have good repeated animal models. Then the good repeated animal model was made from the mice fibrosis cancernoma QR-32. QR-32 cannot proliferate after inoculation in the skin, and will completely disappear; there were no metastasis lump after injecting into the vein. However, if QR-32 was injected with Gelatin sponge together under the skin in the mice, QR-32 will become the proliferating tumor cells QRSP.

In vitro culturing QRSP and then transfer into another mice, even if there is no foreign thing, the tumors will grow such as the lung metastasis will happen after injection in the vein.

$XZ-C_4$ was used in the animal models to search the effects of the tumor development. To divide this animal models into two steps: the process from QR-32 to QRSP(early progress) and from the QRSP to tumor(later progress). After using $XZ-C_4$, the tumor development will be inhibited in these two models, especially the former will be inhibited significantly. And this has relationship with the dose of the medication.

On the survival experiment the animal models of the inoculation of the QR-32 AND Gelatin sponge died during 65 days, however in XZ-C group the mice survival rate for 150 days was 30%. $XZ-C_4$ can increase the immune effects and reduce the side effects of other anticancer medication.

This research proved that $XZ-C_4$ has inhibition of the cancer progression function and inhibit cancer invasion and metastasis.

3). Z-C1+Z-C4 anti-cancer immune regulation medication

Z-C1+Z-C4 anti-cancer immune regulation medication has the following characteristics:
A. An overall improvement in the quality of life of patients with advanced cancer
B. Protect Thymus and increase immune function;
Nurse bone morrow and blood and increase immune function
C. Enhance physical fitness, reduce pain and improve physical strength
D. Enhance therapeutic effect and reduce the side effects of chemotherapy

5. Z-C Medication is the Modern Production of Traditional Herb Medication

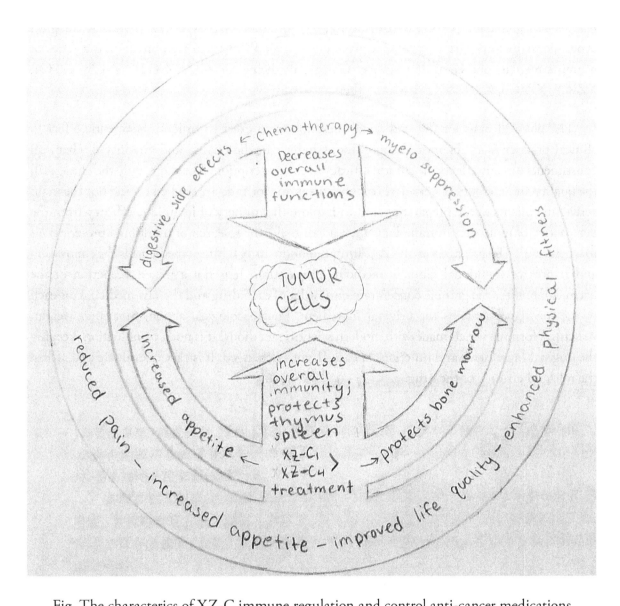

Fig. The characterics of XZ-C immune regulation and control anti-cancer medications

XZ-C immunomodulation anticancer Chinese medicine is not an experience prescription, nor is it an old Chinese medicine practice prescription, but it is the scientific research results of the combination of Chinese and Western medicine and the modernization of traditional Chinese medicine are combined with modern medical methods, experimental tumor research methods and modern pharmacological and pharmacodynamic research methods. After 7 years of more than 4,000 cancer-bearing animal models, 200 commonly used anti-cancer Chinese herbal medicines were screened in animal experiments in batches, and screened for tumor inhibition rates in vitro and in tumor-bearing animals.

48 kinds of traditional Chinese medicines with anti-cancer effects were screened out. Then it was made as these 48 kinds of natural medicines into XZ-C1~10.

According to the respiratory system, digestive system, urinary system, gynecology, endocrine system, the cancer animal models of liver cancer, stomach cancer, colon cancer, breast cancer, bladder cancer and lung cancer were made and the immunological experiments and toxicological experiments in tumor-bearing animals were done, then all of them were made into a series of immune regulate and control anticancer Chinese medicine XZ-C1, XZ-C2, XZ-C3, XZ-C4, XZ-C5, XZ-C6, XZ-C7, XZ-C8 and others.

The physical basis for the traditional prescription to exert its unique therapeutic effect in clinical practice is its chemical composition. Changes in the quality and quantity of chemical constituents directly affects the clinical efficacy of the prescription. Therefore, only the changes in the quality and quantity of chemical components in the formula are studied to find out the main active ingredients of the preparation and to Explore the mystery of its unique efficacy from the perspective of molecular immunology, then it can make the research of traditional prescriptions to a new level. The preparation of XZ-C immunomodulatory Chinese medicine is the innovation and reform of traditional Chinese medicine preparation. It is not a mixed decoction of the chemical, but it is the granule concentrate or powder of each drug and the raw medicine for each of the medicines remains the original ingredient, pharmacological action, molecular weight, structural formula which made with modern scientific methods. It is not a combination, keeping the original ingredients and functions of each flavor unchanged. It is easy to evaluate and affirm the role and efficacy of the drug.

B. The Second Article

Walked out of the new road of cancer therapy with immune regulation and control of the combination of Chinese and western medicine

Strive to follow the path of independent innovation with Chinese characteristics and adhere to walk on the independent innovation road of "Chinese-style anti-cancer" with the combination of Chinese and Western medicine

Walked out of the new road of cancer therapy with immune regulation and control of the combination of Chinese and western medicine

Search or avigate
Path finding and footprint
Walked out of a new road of cancer treatment with XZ-C immune regulation and control of the combination of Chinese and Western medicine at the molecular level
The theory system of cancer treatment with XZ-C immunoregulation and cancer treatment has been formed, which is the theory basis and experimental basis of cancer immunotherapy
A series products and adaptation range of XZ-C immune regulation anti-cancer Chinese medicine
XZ-C immunomodulation anticancer Chinese medicine is the result of the modernization of traditional Chinese medicine

Chapter III

"Walked out of the new road of cancer treatment of immune regulation and control of combination of Chinese and Western medicine"

Walked out of the new road to overcome cancer

Volume II

Experimental research and anti-cancer research of combination of Western medicine and Chinese medicine immunopharmacology at the molecular level

——Walked out of the new way of conquering cancer with XZ-C immune regulation and control of combination of Chinese and western medicine at the molecular level Chinese and Western medicine

——Walked out of the new way of conquering cancer with Chinese medicine immune regulation and control, regulating immune activity, preventing thymus atrophy, promoting thymic hyperplasia, protecting bone marrow hematopoietic function, improving immune surveillance, and combining Western medicine at the molecular level

Contents

First, it has formed the theoretical system of XZ-C immune regulation of cancer treatment and has walked out of the new path of conquering cancer for more than 60 years which is experiencing the clinical application and observation and verification

Second, finding the way

Third, the innovation content of the research theory of the new concepts and the new methods of cancer metastasis therapy

Foreword (1)

Why did I take the title of the book as: "Walked out of a new road of conquering cancer", the title of the book is due to the guidance and inspiration from several experts, scholars, seniors, and teachers.

On July 2, 2001, Academician **Wu Wei** mentioned in his letter: "**The overall impression is: from clinical to experimental, from experimental to clinical mode is very good, the road of combining Chinese and Western medicine is also very correct, I sincerely wish you Keep moving forward and get out of a new path of conquering cancer.**"

On February 22, 2006, **Academician Tang Yu** mentioned in his letter: "... Chinese medicine and biological therapy are the two most promising ways to anti-metastasis, especially Chinese medicine. I hope that you will walk out of the anti-metastasis road with Chinese characteristics."

On March 22, 2006, Academician *Liu Yunyi mentioned in his letter: "...I agree with your concept and thinking about cancer in your book... I hope that you can make a breakthrough contribution to traditional Chinese medicine to make the majority of patients Benefiting, the traditional Chinese medicine can be further developed, and my medical career will reach a world status."*

On January 9, 2006, Academician Wu Xianzhong mentioned in his letter: "...the tumor is a difficult bone, but it should continue to be continued. Fortunately, everyone is very objective, only if it is effective, whether it is treating the tumor or the body. In the letter of April 10, 2012, "We think that the road you have traveled is very special. Methods, drug combinations, and the development of XZ-C series of drugs have all innovated and formed their own patents. This road should continue."

Thanks for their guidance, guidance, and assistance in our research work, research thinking, research direction, research routes, research goals, and research methods. Our research work has been working in the direction of its guidance. I would like to express my gratitude to the academicians Wu Hao, Tang Wei, Wu Xianzhong and Liu Yunyi.

In the past 28 years (1985-present), cancer research has achieved a series of scientific and technological innovations and scientific research achievements in animal experimental research, clinical basic research and clinical verification. After 20 years of hard work, XZ-C immune regulation has been initially formed. Anti-cancer treatment. In the past 20 years, a new road to cancer has been taken out.

In the past 20 years, this series of experimental and clinical research work has received enthusiastic support and cordial guidance from internationally renowned foreign scientists and Chinese general practitioners. In 1990, when the author submitted the "Eighth Five-Year Plan" key scientific and technological research project to the State Science and Technology Commission (to further explore the anti-cancer and anti-metastasis experimental and clinical studies of cancer and anti-cancer Chinese herbal medicine for precancerous lesions of liver cancer and gastrointestinal cancer), Academician Yan said in an expert opinion: "It is a very important topic to study cancer metastasis and how to prevent metastasis. It is feasible to explore clinical prevention methods through experimental research and it is beneficial to people's work." Under the guidance of my teacher, rigorous academics, and scientific study, we have initially completed the above projects, and I would like to thank you.

Scientific research must have nutritional feeding of the literature. In 1986, we just established an experimental surgical animal laboratory to make an animal model of cancer metastasis and conduct experimental research. We saw Professor Gao Jin's book "Invasion and Metastasis of Cancer - Basic Research and Clinical Medicine", and saw the monograph of Academician Tang Wei, "Basic and Clinical Metastasis and Recurrence of Liver Cancer". The theories in the two books make us suddenly clear. It also encourages and promotes our experimental work and clinical validation work from another aspect. Professor Tang Wei proposed in his monograph: "The **The next important goal of primary liver cancer research is prevention and treatment of recurrence and metastasis, and said: "metastasis and recurrence have become a bottleneck to further improve the survival rate of liver cancer, and are one of the most important difficulties in combating cancer." It gives us the wisdom and courage to update our thinking and be brave in innovation. It also strengthens the confidence and determination of our experimental team. I would like to express my gratitude to Academician Tang Wei and Professor Gao Jin.** I would like to express my gratitude to Academician Tang Wei and Professor Gao Jin.

In the past 7 years, we have used more than 6,000 tumor-bearing animal models to explore one basic problem after another. The screening of 200 kinds of Chinese herbal medicines in the tumor-bearing animal model in vivo was carried out by several graduate students. Master Zhu Siping, Dr. Zou Shaomin, Master Li Zhengxun, Master of Liu Wei, etc., they carried out and completed a lot of hard work. The experimental work, hard work, day and night, contributed to the development of experimental oncology medicine for anti-cancer and anti-cancer. I sincerely thank you all.

Foreword (2)

Experimental surgery is extremely important in the development of medicine. It is a key to open the medical exclusion zone. Many disease prevention methods have been studied in many animal experiments, and the stability results have been applied to the clinic to promote the development of the medical cause.

Developing science and technological innovation, the laboratory is the key condition. I deeply understand the importance of the laboratory. I am the first batch of college students in the post-liberation college entrance examination. I have not studied or studied abroad, but I have achieved many international achievements. The key is that I have a good laboratory. In the 1960s, I participated in the open heart surgery laboratory for cardiopulmonary bypass. In the 1980s, I established a cirrhosis ascites laboratory. In the 1990s, I established the Institute of Experimental Surgery to focus on cancer. My animal laboratory has good equipment conditions, including white mice, white rats, Dutch pigs, rabbits, dogs, monkeys and other animal experiments. It has a good sterilization operating room and can be used for major surgery and animals in the chest and abdomen. After the postoperative observation room, various designs, ideas, and experimental operations can be used to achieve results or conclusions.

Therefore, the laboratory is the key condition, and the key is to build a good equipment laboratory.

University teachers should have dual tasks on their shoulders. One is to do a good job of teaching; the other is to develop science.

University teachers should have good laboratories for scientific research, follow the scientific development concept, base on known science, explore unknown science, face the future science, emerging disciplines, marginal disciplines, interdisciplinary, face the frontiers of science, strive for innovation, advancement, The hall of science, adding bricks and tiles.

In summary, experimental research and basic research are very important. Without experimental research and breakthroughs in basic research, clinical efficacy is difficult to improve, and it is difficult to propose new understandings, new concepts, and new theoretical insights. Among them, the experiment is the key. I have a good laboratory. I am the director of the Institute of Experimental Surgery and the director of clinical surgery. The experimental research, basic research and clinical verification are easy to take care of.

Basic research in medicine is very important for achieving progress in combating diseases. Experimental oncology is the basic science of cancer prevention research and has promoted the continuous development of cancer research in China.

Our Experimental Surgery Institute conducted a series of experimental studies to explore the mechanisms of cancer onset, invasion and recurrence and metastasis. We conducted a full-scale experimental study of tumors in the laboratory for 4 years. From experimental tumor research, we found that thymus atrophy and immune function are low. May be the cause of the tumor, one of the pathogenesis, how to prevent thymus atrophy? How to regulate immune function is low? How to promote immunity? How to "protect the chest"? Immune regulation should be carried out, and Western medicine should be combined at the molecular level to embark on a new path of Chinese characteristics to overcome cancer.

Facing the future of medicine, we will look forward to the future. After 60 years of hard work, we will practice the scientific development concept and face the frontier of science, striving for innovation and progress. To overcome cancer, we must come from the clinical, through experimental research, to the clinical, to solve the actual problems of patients; must seek truth from facts, use facts, use data to speak; must constantly self-transcend, self-advance; in scientific research should emancipate the mind, Breaking away the traditional old ideas, based on independent innovation and original innovation; our research route for decades is to find problems → ask questions → study problems → solve problems or explain problems, the road is like this, step by step, difficult trek, we hope Stepping out of an innovative road of anti-cancer and anti-transfer with Chinese characteristics and independent intellectual property rights.

Our research on oncology medical research is based on patients, discovering and asking questions from clinical work, conducting in-depth basic research on animal experiments, and then turning basic research results into clinical applications to improve the overall level of medical care and ultimately benefit patients.

First, Walked out of the new way of cancer treatment with immune regulation and control of the combination of Chinese and Western medicine

Volume II

Experimental research and anti-cancer research of combination of Western medicine and Chinese medicine immunopharmacology at the molecular level

——Walked out of the new way of conquering cancer with XZ-C immune regulation and control of combination of Chinese and western medicine at the molecular level Chinese and Western medicine

——Walked out of thenew way of conquering cancer with Chinese medicine immune regulation and control, regulating immune activity, preventing thymus atrophy, promoting thymic hyperplasia, protecting bone marrow hematopoietic function, improving immune surveillance, and combining Western medicine at the molecular level

1. New findings in anti-cancer and anti-cancer metastasis research

Implications of anti-cancer metastasis

I am a clinical surgeon. Why do you study cancer? This is due to the results of the patient interviews with a group of cancer patients.

In 1985, I conducted a petition with more than 3,000 patients with postoperative chest and abdominal cancer. The results showed that most of the patients relapsed or metastasized 2-3 years after surgery, and some even after several months and one year after surgery. Recurrence and metastasis.

From the follow-up results, it was found that postoperative recurrence and metastasis were the key factors affecting the long-term efficacy of surgery.

Therefore, we also raised an important issue: clinicians must pay attention to and study the prevention and treatment of postoperative recurrence and metastasis, in order to improve the long-term efficacy of postoperative. Therefore, it is necessary to conduct an experimental study of the clinical basis of recurrence and metastasis. Without a breakthrough in basic research, clinical efficacy is difficult to improve.

So we established the Experimental Surgery Laboratory (later established the Experimental Surgery Research Institute of Hubei College of Traditional Chinese Medicine in 1991, the research direction is to overcome cancer).

We have carried out research from the following two aspects: one is animal experimental research: one is clinical research. Based on the success of animal experiments, it is applied clinically for clinical validation. After 60 years of hard work, a series of experimental research and clinical verification work were carried out, and a series of scientific and technological innovations were obtained.

New discovery

(1) From the results of follow-up, it was found that:

1. postoperative recurrence and metastasis are the key factors affecting the long-term efficacy of surgery.
2. clinicians must pay attention to and study the prevention and treatment measures for postoperative recurrence and metastasis.

(2) From the experimental tumor research, it was found that:

1) Excision of the thymus (Thymus, TH) can be used to create a model of cancer-bearing animals. Injection of immunosuppressive agents can also contribute to the establishment of animal models of cancer-bearing animals. The conclusion of the study clearly proves

that the occurrence and development of cancer has a clear positive relationship with the host immune organ TH and immune organ tissue function. It is difficult to manufacture animal models without removing the TH. Repeated experiments repeatedly confirmed the experimental results.

2) Whether it is immune first and then easy to get cancer or cancer first and then low immunity, our experimental results are: first, there is low immunity and then easy to have cancer, the development, if no immune function decline, it is not easy to vaccinate successfully. The results of this study suggest that improving and maintaining good immune function and protecting the thymus of the immune organs is one of the important measures to prevent cancer.

3) The animal model of liver metastasis was established in our laboratory to study the relationship between metastasis and immunity in cancer. Group A and B were divided into groups. Group A used immunosuppressants, and group B was different. The result was that the number of intrahepatic metastases in group A was significantly higher than that in group B. The results of this experiment suggest that metastasis is associated with immunity, low immune function or the use of immunosuppressive agents may promote tumor metastasis.

4) Our laboratory conducted an experiment to investigate the effects of tumors on the immune organs of the body. It was found that the thymus was progressively atrophied as the cancer progressed. Immediately after inoculation of cancer cells, the thymus of the host showed acute progressive atrophy, cell proliferation was blocked, and the volume was significantly reduced. The results of this experiment suggest that the tumor will inhibit the thymus and cause the immune organs to shrink.

5) Through experiments we also found that some experimental mice were not vaccinated, or the tumor grew very small, the thymus did not significantly shrink, in order to understand the relationship between tumor and thymus atrophy, so we experimented in a group of experimental mice transplanted solid tumors to grow When the thumb is large, it is removed. After 1 month, the thymus was found to have no progressive atrophy. Therefore, we speculate that a solid tumor may produce a factor that is not known to inhibit the thymus, which needs further study.

6) The above experimental results prove that the progression of the tumor causes the thymus to undergo atrophy. Then, can we adopt some methods to prevent the host thymus from shrinking. Therefore, we further designed and wanted to use this immune organ cell transplantation to restore the experimental function of the immune organ. Our laboratory is investigating the atrophy of the thymus gland in suppressing tumor progression, looking for ways to restore the function of the thymus and reconstituting the immune system. Experimental study on the immune function of fetal liver, fetal spleen and fetal thymocyte transplantation in mice. The results showed that: S, T, L three groups of cells combined transplantation, the recent complete tumor regression rate was 40%, the long-term tumor complete regression rate was 46.67%, and the tumor disappeared long-term survival.

7) When we explored the effect of tumor on the spleen of the immune organs of the body, we found that the spleen has an inhibitory effect on tumor growth in the early stage of the tumor, and in the late stage of the tumor, the spleen also shows progressive atrophy. The results of this study suggest that the spleen has a bidirectional effect on tumor growth, which has a certain inhibitory effect in the early stage and loses its inhibitory effect in the late stage. Spleen cell transplantation can enhance the inhibition of tumors. This is a new discovery in experimental research and is a very important finding that should be further studied.

In summary, from the above series of experimental studies, it is found that thymus atrophy, immune dysfunction may be one of the causes and pathogenesis of cancer, and should further from the function and tissue structure of the thymus, immune function is low and how to promote immunity, so that immune reconstruction, How to protect your chest from further research, review the structure of the thymus and the function of the thymus, and find new ways and means of cancer treatment.

In summary, from the above series of experimental studies, found that thymus atrophy, immune dysfunction may be one of the causes and pathogenesis of cancer, and should further from the function and organization of the thymus, Low immune function and how to promote immunity, make immune reconstruction, How to protect the thymus and to increase immune function from further research. Let's review the structure of the thymus and the function of the thymus to find new ways and means of cancer treatment.

Experimental research

---

2. Experimental observation of the influence of tumor on the thymus of immune organs

It is generally believed that the immune function of the body affects the occurrence, development and prognosis of the tumor, and the tumor also has an inhibitory effect on the immune state of the body. The two are causal and intricate. In the animal experiment of the effect of spleen on tumor growth, the author observed that many changes occurred in the thymus and spleen of the immune organs of tumor-bearing mice. It seems that there is a certain regularity **in order to further explore the relationship between the tumor and the spleen and thymus and its regularity. The following experiments were designed to dynamically observe the changes in the conversion rate of thymus, spleen and lymphocytes in tumor-bearing mice at different times to explore the regularity between them.**

【Materials and Methods】

(1) Experimental animals and grouping

40 Kunming mice were randomly divided into 4 groups, aged 40~50d, weighing 15~18g. Male or female.

Group I: healthy control group, healthy mice that were not inoculated with cancer cells, and the thymus, spleen and peripheral blood were taken for observation after sacrifice.

Group II: 0.1×10^7 Ehrlich ascites tumor cells were inoculated intraperitoneally, and sacrificed after 3 days.

Group III: Inoculated tumor cells (ibid.), and sacrificed on the 7th day.

Group IV: Observation on the 14th day of inoculation of tumor cells.

Take the experiment in the previous (the experimental study on the effect of spleen on tumor growth). The results of autopsy after 100 natural deaths in tumor-bearing mice, as a result of changes in thymus and spleen of advanced tumor, thymus in late stage tumor-bearing mice The average diameter is (1.2 ± 0.3) mm, the average weight is (20 ± 5) mg, and the texture is hard. The spleen is extremely atrophied, with an average weight of (60 ± 12) mg. The texture is hard, the color is gray, the growth center is significantly reduced, and fibrosis occurs.

(2) Experimental method

Each group of mice was sacrificed by excretion of the eyeball at the scheduled time. Each mouse was given 1 ml of whole blood (heparin anticoagulation) for lymphocyte transformation test, and then the mice were immediately dissected to observe the tumor. Infiltration range, ascites volume and the involvement of various organs, and the anatomy of the thymus, spleen and lymph nodes were observed with the naked eye. The thymus and spleen were completely removed, and the volume was measured with a vernier caliper.

[Experimental results]

(1) The weight of thymus at different stages after inoculation of tumor cells in mice is shown in Table 1.

Perform variance analysis on Table 1, see Table 2. The results of Tables 1 and 2 are shown by curves, and the thymus weight change curve (Fig. 1) is plotted. The weight of the thymus on the 25th and 30th days in the figure is from the experimental results in the previous data.

1. Comparison of thymus weights of mice in each group (mg)

Group	normal group I	group II 3 days after vaccination group		group III 7 days after vaccination	group IV 14 days after vaccination
X_{ij}	72.8	78.2		90.0	40.0
	50.0	83.4		66.0	32.2
	56.4	89		85.4	39.8
	96.4	68		106.5	23.5
	77.4	74.8		51.7	38.0
	100.7	95.4		77.8	36.0
	87.5	11.50		73	46.0
	76.8	56.4		60	20.0
	112.7	43.0		49.4	55
	51.0				20
ΣX	781.07	703.2	736.3	350.5	ΣX 2 571.7
N_i	10	9	10	10	N 39
$\_Xi$	78.17	78.13	73.63	35.05	$\_X$ 65.94
$\Sigma_i X^2$	6 6261.79	58 566.66	57 033.75	18 467.25	ΣX^2 191 324.75

Table 2 Analysis of variance for Table 1

Source of variation	SS	V	MS	F	P
Between Groups	12 967.10	3	4 322.36	12.85	<0.01
Within Groups	11 777.12	35	336.48		
Total	24 744.22	38			

As can be seen from Table 1, Table 2, and Figure 1, the thymus of the tumor-bearing mice showed a regular change. Within 7 days after inoculation, there was no significant change in the thymus macroscopic view, but the weight had begun to decrease. After the day, it is acute progressive atrophy. The diameter of each leaf of the late thymus is reduced from the normal 5~8mm to about 1mm, the weight is reduced from 76.1mg to 20mg, the texture becomes hard, and the function is also reduced or even lost. It shows that the cellular immune function of the body is increasingly manipulated and inhibited as the tumor progresses, causing the immune function to be low and the tumor to grow faster and faster.

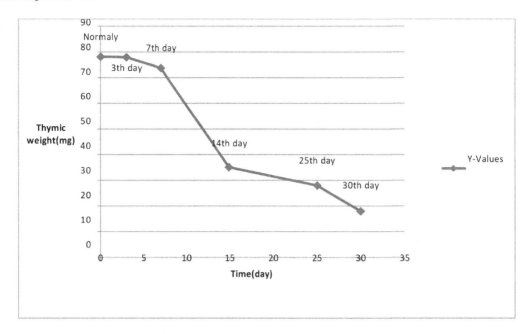

Figure 1 the curve of variation on the thymic weights

(2) Pathological changes in the thymus

Thymus: progressive atrophy throughout the course of the disease. On the third day after inoculation of the tumor cells, the thymus was slightly shrunk and the color was slightly gray. On the 7th day after inoculation, the thymus volume was significantly atrophied, cell proliferation was blocked, and mature cells were reduced. By the end of the tumor, the thymus is extremely atrophied, the volume is about the size of sesame seeds, the diameter is 1mm, and the texture becomes hard.

(3) About the impact of tumor on the thymus

The experimental results show that after inoculation of the tumor cells, the thymus is immediately suppressed, and the whole process is progressively atrophy, so the thymus quickly loses the anti-tumor immune effect. It was observed in the experiment that the thymus gland changed its morphological structure shortly after inoculation of the tumor cells, and the whole course of disease showed progressive atrophy. By the end of the tumor, the weight of the thymus was reduced from 78.13±13.2 mg to 20±5 mg, and the volume was reduced from 5 to 8 mm in diameter to 1 mm. Cell proliferation was significantly blocked.

Due to progressive atrophy of the thymus, cell proliferation is blocked, mature cells are reduced or depleted, the index is decreased, metabolism is weakened, cell viability is decreased, and thymus hormone secretion is also reduced. The cellular immune function of the body is inevitably damaged, and the defense ability of the mouse is low. The transplanted cancer cells grow and multiply. Zhang Tongwen and other similar reports have found that the thymus atrophy of tumor-bearing mice is accompanied by the inhibition of bone marrow cell proliferation and the decrease of nucleated cell viability, and it is considered

that there is a close relationship between the two. It can be seen that the inhibition or damage effect of the tumor on the host immune function is multifaceted, affecting the entire immune system of the body. This group of lymphocyte transformation rate test showed that after inoculation of cancer cells, the lymphocyte transformation rate showed a progressive decline, and decreased to more than 50% in the late stage, indicating that the cellular immune effect was inhibited. As for why the thymus of tumor-bearing mice is inhibited and atrophied, further experimental research and observation are needed.

The thymus also produces a variety of thymus hormones that promote the differentiation and maturation of immune lymphocyte stem cells. Although the thymus is a lymphoid organ, due to the presence of the blood thymus barrier, the thymus does not directly interact with the antigenic substance to exert an effect. Thus, it is not proliferated by the stimulation of tumor-specific antigens. The tumor produces secretory immunosuppressive factors that act on the thymus, causing progressive atrophy and functional damage.

For Immunotherapy for malignant tumors, many doctors are committed to the development of this field with great interest.

Since the 1980s, due to the rapid development of immunology and biotechnology, it has provided an opportunity for immunotherapy for cancer patients. The theory of biological response regulation has been proposed, and a fourth therapeutic program other than surgery, radiotherapy, and chemotherapy has been established. That is, tumor biotherapy (BRM). The use of biological modulators to treat tumors may be promising for the development of new therapies for effective immunotherapy for tumors.

In short, the host and the tumor are a contradiction, and have existed throughout the process of tumor development and development. In the case of a healthy function of the body's immune system, the body can restrict and destroy tumors through its cellular and humoral immune responses. On the other hand, the growing tumor has a lot of effects on the body's immune system, inhibiting the body's immune function and promoting the development of the tumor.

3. Morphology and location of the thymus

The thymus (thymus) is a cone-shaped shape, which can be divided into two leaves that are not symmetrical to the left and right. The texture is soft and long and flat, and the two leaves are connected by connective tissue (Fig. A). The size of the thymus varies greatly from age to age. In the late embryonic development and neonates, the growth rate of the thymus is very fast. From birth to 2 years old, it is the best period for thymus development, weighing 15-20g. With the increase of age, the thymus continues to grow, but it is relatively slower than the post-natal period, reaching 25~40g in puberty. After puberty, the thymus begins to shrink and degenerate. The adult thymus still retains its original shape, but its structure changes greatly, lymphocytes are greatly reduced, and thymus tissue is often replaced by adipose tissue.

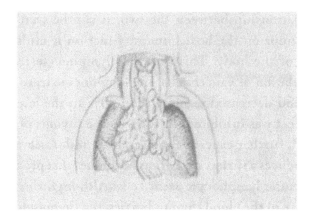

Figure A Morphological location of the thymus in children

The adult thymus is in the anterior portion of the mediastinum behind the sternum. The posterior is adjacent to the innominate vein and the aortic arch, and the sides are adjacent to the mediastinal pleura and lung. Thymial enlargement and thymoma can compress the above organs and have corresponding clinical symptoms.

The thymus of the child is large in volume, the upper end can extend to the base of the neck, some can reach the lower edge of the thyroid, and the lower end can extend into the anterior mediastinum to reach the front of the pericardium.

4. The structure of the thymus

(1) Capsule: The thymus surface is covered with a connective tissue film, and the film is composed of a dense collagen fiber bundle, an elastic fiber, and a matrix. The connective tissue fiber bundle in the capsule protrudes into the thymus parenchyma and divides the thymus into many leaflets. The periphery of the lobules is the cortex, and the deep side is the medulla. There is a scaffold composed of reticular epithelial cells (Fig. as the following).

(2) Cortex: The cortex of the thymus is located in the periphery of the leaflet and consists of dense lymphocytes and epithelial reticular cells. Lymphocytes in the superficial cortex are larger and belong to the original lymphocyte type. The middle layer of lymphocytes is medium in size, and the inner layer is mostly small linba cells. There are scattered macrophages in the cortex. From shallow to deep is the process by which hematopoietic stem cells proliferate and differentiate into T lymphocytes.

(3) Medulla: The medulla of the thymus is located deep in the leaflet and consists of epithelial reticular cells and a small number of lymphocytes. There are scattered thymus bodies in the medulla. The body is round or oval, consisting of several layers of epithelium(Fig. as the following)

Figure 2. Upper mediastinal organ and pericardium and thymus in adult
T: thymus; L: lung; H: heart

Figure 3 Structure of the thymus in children
1, small leaf interval; 2, thymus lobules; 3, thymus on the mass; 4, thymus small body; 5, the capsule; 6, medulla; 7, keratinized epithelial cells and debris; 8, epithelial cells; 9, thymocytes

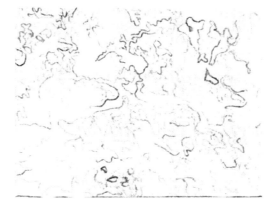

Figure 4. Thymic medulla
The scattered thymus bodies (arrows) distributed in the medulla

Thymus function

The function of the thymus is complex, the thymus is a lymphoid organ, and has the function of an endocrine gland. Some authors have included it in the endocrine system. **Its main function is to cultivate and manufacture T lymphocytes and secrete thymus hormone.** The cultivation of T cells in the thymus requires a suitable internal environment. The epithelial network of the thymus can secrete a variety of hormones: thymosin, thymopoietin, thymulin, thymic humoral factor (THF), and ubiguitin. These hormones together with macrophages and staggered cells in the thymus form a microenvironment for culturing T cells. Thymosin and thymosin can promote the differentiation of lymphocyte stem cells into T-cells, stimulate T cell proliferation, and stimulate the hypothalamic secretion of ACTH and LH; Thymogenin induces T cell differentiation; other hormones promote synergistic effects on early division of T cells and promotion of T cell maturation.

Primitive lymphatic stem cells have no immunity and are further developed into T cells with immune function. Then through the blood circulation to the surrounding lymphoid organs, such as lymphoid tissue, lymph nodes, spleen, etc., after antigen activation and proliferation, participate in the immune response. Although the adult thymus is atrophied and degraded, it still has the ability to secrete thymus hormone. When the lymphoid tissue of the body is destroyed, the T cells are greatly reduced, and the lymphatic stem cells that enter the thymus with blood circulation can still be converted into T cells under the action of thymus hormone.

T lymphocyte

Differentiation and development of lymphocytes in the thymus

Phenotypic changes during T cell differentiation and development

It is currently known that the main factors inducing differentiation and maturation of T cells in the thymus include: 1 Thymic stromal cells (TSC) interact directly with thymocytes via adhesion molecules on the cell surface; 2 Thymic stromal cells secrete a variety of cytokines (such as IL-1, IL-6, IL-7) and thymus hormone to induce thymocyte differentiation; 3 Thymocytes secrete a variety of cytokines (such as IL-2, IL-4) also play an important role in the differentiation and maturation of thymocytes themselves. In addition, thymic epithelial cells, macrophages, and dendritic cells play a decisive role in self-tolerance, MHC restriction, and formation of T cell function subpopulations during thymocyte differentiation.

A T cell, or T lymphocyte, is called T cells because they mature in Thymus from thymocytes (although some also mature in the tonsils) and All T cells originate from haematopoietic stem cells in the bone marrow. In the bone marrow haematopoietic stem cells become haematopoietic progenitors; on the way to thymus haematopoietic progenitors are expanded by cell division to generate a large population of immature thymocytes; is a type of lymphocyte (a subtype of white blood cell) that plays a central role in cell-mediated immunity.

T cells can be distinguished from other lymphocytes by the presence of a T-cell receptor on the cell surface. There are several subsets of T cells, each of which has a distinct function such as Cytotoxic (Killer) or CD8+T cells, helper T cells or CD4+ T cells, Natural killer T cells, etc. Two distinct types of thymocytes are produced in the thymus: CD4/CD8. in the thymus the earlist thymocytes are double- negative (CD4-CD8-) cells, later become double-positive thymocytes (CD4+CD8+); finally mature to single-positive (CD4+CD8- or CD4-CD8+) thymocytes. About 98% of thymocytes die during the development processes in the thymus by failing either positive selection or negative selection, whereas 2% matured naïve T cells leave the thymus and begin to spread throughout the body, including the lymph nodes. As the thymus shrinks by about 3% a year throughout middle age, there is a corresponding fall in the thymic production of naive T cells, leaving peripheral T cell expansion to play a greater role in protecting older subjects.

5. the body's immune function

In particular, the function of cellular immunity and T lymphocytes gradually decreases with age, and the thymus gradually degenerates in structure and function after adulthood. The thymus is the central organ of immune function and is the base for differentiation and maturation of T lymphocytes. Thymus epithelial cells produce and release thymosin, which plays an important role in the differentiation of precursor T lymphocytes into mature immune active T cells. The thymus is also the earliest organ of body degradation. It begins to shrink after sexual maturity, and its ability to produce and secrete thymosin gradually decreases with age.

The study of the thymus began in the early 1960s when it was found to be closely related to immune function. Miller et al. (1960) found that immune function dysplasia in dethymocytes (neonatal mice) significantly reduced the number of circulating T cells. For 50 years, the thymus has been recognized as the central organ of the animal's immune system, and is the earliest organ of the body's development. When it matures, the structure and function of the thymus reach a peak, and then gradually shrinks and degenerates with age. Immune function is gradually replaced by spleen and other lymphatic tissue in adult animals. The thymus is the core tissue of T lymphocyte development, and is the base for producing various immune factors (lymphokines, cytokines). Thymosin or thymosin peptide is the main secretory immune regulator. Now there are various thymosin (peptide). The product is used for clinical and experimental research. There are special journals abroad called "thymus", which regularly publish reports on thymus research and clinical treatment.

6. Thymus immune regulation function and NIM theory

From the early days that it is independent from the regulation of other physiological systems of the single automatic control system, the development has considered the thymus and the neuroendocrine system is the function network system with harmonization of interrelated functions. Since the late 1970s, Besedovsky (in 1977) proposed neuroendocrine

immune network theory (NIM), has been recognized as the thymus and immune function is to guide the core idea. Thymus and peripheral nervous system and the immune system response functions is formed of three line contact. The central cerebral cortex, hypothalamus, and pituitary gland are superior regulatory centers; peripheral lymphoid organs and tissues, lymphocytes and cytokines are the regulatory and executive units of the lower or subordinate immune network; the intermediate hub is the thymus, which can be called the middle line of NIM. The path of NIM can be divided into three sections: 1 down line, that is, the central down to the middle line and the lower line; 2 up line, the cytokine feedback information from the lower line to the central part; 3 intermediate line path to The thymus is the main axis, with spleen and other lymphoid tissues and bone marrow progenitor cells. Recent studies have shown that the thymus plays an important role in NIM activities. For example, Fabres (1983) put forward - the concept of "thymic neuroendocrine network", Goldstein AL (1983) that "neuroendocrine - thymus axis" of thought, expression can be described as a special significance in the thymus NIM network.

The thymus begins to degenerate after sexual maturity, and the secreted thymosin and other hormones are also reduced, which hinders the differentiation of T lymphocytes and reduces the immune function of the body. The main cause of aging in humans and mammals is closely related to thymic atrophy and degeneration.

As the age increases, the thymus naturally shrinks and life gradually ages. The thymus is an important factor affecting the body's immune level. Experiments have shown that removal of the thymus from adult rats (2 months old) can accelerate their autoimmune function and aging. At 6 months after thymus surgery in rats (2 months old), the immune activity of spleen lymphocytes decreased significantly, only 51.6% of the same age without thymus.

7. Thymus exocrine function

Thymus hormone activity can be detected by bioassay. Experiments show that the activity of thymus hormone decreases with age, and decreases with thymus atrophy. It is not detected in the serum of animals with thymus removed. The thymus is the main producing area of thymus hormone. Thymosin is a hormone substance secreted by thymocytes and has the effect of regulating immune function.

The thymus is an important tissue of the body's immune function, secreting and producing thymosin (thymulin and other hormones), and secreting IL-1 and IL-2 and other interleukins to regulate the intrinsic function and cell viability of the thymus. At the same time, it is secreted by the pituitary. Adjustment. It can be seen that the research on thymus immunoregulation has provided preliminary evidence that exogenous endocrine hormones (such as prolactin, growth hormone, thyroxine, etc.) can induce the regenerative thymus to regain vitality and maintain immune regulation. **Thymic recession can be reversed, which is the common research and development prospect of modern immunology and endocrinology.**

8. Effect of chemical drugs on the body's immune function

Cyclophosphamide (Cy) or hydrocortisone (HC) is a commonly used drug in clinical practice, which can cause a decline in immune function. Long-term injection can cause atrophy of thymus, spleen and lymph nodes, and significantly reduce immune function.

In short, although Cy and HC have certain inhibitory effects on immune function, such as Cy for 3w, the thymus has shrunk, the spleen begins to shrink after 6w, and the proliferative power of peripheral blood T lymphocytes decreases significantly at 6-12w.

The research of raditional Chinese medicine immunopharmacology

---

9. The naming and function of thymus hormone

Since the early 1960s, the well-known scientists Good and Miller first reported that the function of the thymus is the "central" organ of the systemic immune system, and cellular immunology has developed rapidly. In the early 1970s, a hypothesis about thymus secreting hormones was proposed. Several "presumptive" but not yet confirmed thymosin or hormone-like components were successively introduced. They are peptide components extracted from the whole thymus. Recent studies have shown that thymic epidermal cells (TEC) are cells that produce thymus hormone components and can be divided into two major categories: interleukins (Ils) and thymosin. Foreign studies have shown that there are four thymus hormones: (1) thymosin-α; (2) thymulin; (3) thymopoietin; (4) thymichumoral factor (THF). Thymulin is a 9-peptide binding component that requires zinc binding to be biologically active. The thymus component is extracted from the bovine thymus in foreign countries.

10, immune regulation and immune promoter

In the current situation, immune promoters can be divided into several categories depending on the source.

The first class of immunostimulants is first derived from microbial components.

The fungal glucan containing β-1,3-glucosamine chains has been shown to have a good clinical effect. They promote MΦ killing of bacteria and tumor cells and induce the release of cellular mono-kinks such as interleukin-1 (IL-1), tumor necrosis factor (TNF), colony stimulating factor (CSF), and the like.

The second major class of immune boosters is the thymus extract.

Peptide components are extracted from animal thymus. Various products have been produced in various countries (including China), and all have immunological pharmacological activities, also known as thymus hormones. Zinc thymulin complex is an active component secreted by thymic epithelial cells. Other kinds of thymus crude extracts have clinical effects. Their main function is to enhance the activity of T cells in vivo, but it has no effect on producing new T cells. . In other words, activation of T cells can enhance the body against microbial pathogens, anti-tumor activity and delay the decline of immune function in aging animals. Clinically used for the treatment of chronic infectious diseases and tumors.

The third major class of immunostimulating agents was the recombination cytokine that was developed in the 1980s. These bioactive factors have achieved significant benefits in clinical treatment, the most prominent of which are rIFN-r, rIFN-α, IL-2 (IL-1 to IL-2), TNF, rCSF (such as GM-CSF). This can be said to be a major innovation or breakthrough in immunopharmacology. Recently, monoclonal antibodies (Mabs) and human gene antibodies (H-Ab) have emerged. These new components can be summarized as recombinant peptide immunological substances.

The purification of the above various immunostimulating substances has made remarkable progress, and a variety of effective products have been available, and there are not many chemical substances that have been proven to have clinical therapeutic effects.

11. Research progress on anticancer immune pharmacology of traditional Chinese medicine polysaccharides

Antitumor Study of Lycium Barbarum Polysaccharide, Polyporus Polysaccharide, Lycium Polysaccharide, Lentinus Polysaccharide, Yunzhi and Ganoderma Lucidum Polysaccharides and Tremella Polysaccharide

Mechanism and prospect of anti-tumor effect of polysaccharide drugs

Advances in anti-cancer immunity of traditional Chinese medicine polysaccharides, polysaccharides can improve the body's immune surveillance system including natural killer cells (NK), macrophages (MΦ), killer T cells (CTL), T cells, LAK cells, tumor infiltrating lymphocytes (TIL)), the activity of interleukin (IL) and other cytokines to achieve the purpose of killing tumor cells. Although many polysaccharides have a certain anti-tumor effect, the two immunopotentiators, including the two polysaccharides, have higher therapeutic effects, and the polysaccharide can be further improved by the same treatment as chemotherapy or radiotherapy.

Research overview and progress

Thomas and Burnet's immunosurveillance theory suggests that the in vivo immune system has the effect of eliminating tumor cells produced by cell mutations in order to maintain a single cell type of each cell. The body's immune surveillance system for tumors includes cellular and humoral immunity, and cellular immunity is particularly important for tumor rejection. Immune cells that perform cellular immune functions include natural killer cells (NK) and macrophages (MΦ). Recently, LAK cells and tumor infiltrating lymphocytes (TIL) have been proposed. The anti-tumor effect of the latter is 50-100 stronger than that of LAK cells. Double, played a stronger role. If these effector cells are inhibited, it is difficult to function as an immunosurveillance system. Elston reported that only 19 patients with choriocarcinoma with cellular immune response died, while 13 patients with no immune response or significantly reduced immune response had 13 deaths, indicating that the level of immune function plays an important role in tumor therapy. . Prevention and treatment of tumors by enhancing the body's immune function is undoubtedly a research field with bright prospects.

According to the research progress of polysaccharides at home and abroad and related information, polysaccharides including LBP can play the role of antibacterial, antiviral, antitumor, anti-aging, anti-chemotherapy side effects and anti-autoimmune diseases on the one hand; There may also be various physiological activities such as lowering blood pressure, lowering blood fat, anti-vomiting, and lowering blood stasis. These aspects will also be an important direction for LBP's in-depth research and application development.

Compared with other polysaccharides, LBP is a glycopeptide with strong action, small dosage, good water solubility, stability and easy absorption by oral administration. It can be considered as a highly effective immune T cell adjuvant. However, LBP is still a crude extract. It is still to be cooperated with phytochemical experts to purify and modify LBP including degradation of oligosaccharides and oligosaccharides with different molecular weights and sulfated polysaccharides. It is expected to further enhance the immunological activity of LBP in order to find a newer, immunologically active drug.

Immunization is closely related to aging. Many scholars have further discovered that the main cause of the deterioration of cellular immune function during aging is that the thymus shrinks with age. It is suggested that the thymus is the biological clock that controls immune function during aging. LBP is the main link in aging immunity - the thymus. The main experiments are as follows: 1 LBP mainly chooses to act on thymic T cells; 2 Ding Yan et al report that LBP can promote the increase of the number of thymic mature T cells, and enhance the "empty" function, so that thymocytes metastasize to the periphery and play the thymus. Immune center regulation, enhance the role of resistance to disease and delay aging; 3 Our experiments have shown that aged mice drink LBP aqueous solution daily, after six months, the control group thymus atrophy, LBP group thymus atrophy recovery, weight increase, but Not yet reached the normal level of adulthood. This fact suggests that LBP can reverse the retrograde thymic degeneration. Based on the above, it is clear that the thymus is related to aging.

12. Characteristics of traditional Chinese medicine immunopharmacology

Compared with Western medicine immunopharmacology, traditional Chinese medicine immunopharmacology has its own characteristics or advantages, and each has its own shortcomings. The advantages of traditional Chinese medicine immunology are as follows:

First of all, long-term clinical managers have accumulated a large number of prescriptions to regulate the body's immune function, especially the beneficial Chinese medicines generally have the effect of regulating immune activity.

Traditional Chinese medicine is rich in sources. In recent years, research has increasingly proved that traditional Chinese medicine is an effective medicine for long-term clinical treatment. After extraction, it can obtain obvious pharmacological effects (including immunomodulatory effects), and the research process saves people time and has high efficiency.

Secondly, traditional Chinese medicines, whether single-agent or prescription, contain multiple active ingredients, unlike Western medicine (synthetic drugs), which are single-structured substances. The role of traditional Chinese medicine is multifaceted. In addition to regulating immune function, it has a certain effect on the whole functional system and organs. And these roles are connected and combined.

The role of traditional Chinese medicine in regulating immune function is generally beneficial, that is, within the normal adjustment range, two-way regulation is the main feature. The tonic drug can be called immunomodulatory drugs, causing a non-specific immune response.

Chinese medicines for tonics have the function of regulating the immune function of the body. Under the general experimental conditions, the correlation between dose and benefit is presented, especially in normal healthy animal experiments. When the animal is at a low level of immune activity (such as dethymus, aging animals or chemotherapy drugs cyclophosphamide inhibition and tumor animals), the tonic drugs improve the body's immunity is more significant.

Immunopharmacology is an interdisciplinary subject formed by the combination of immunology and pharmacology. Traditional Chinese medicine immunopharmacology plays a special important role in immunopharmacology in China. Traditional Chinese medicine immunopharmacology can be understood as a new discipline in the grafting of traditional Chinese medicine and modern immunopharmacology.

As early as the 1970s, Professor Zhou Jin had been calling for the establishment of pharmacology in the integration of Chinese and Western medicine in China, and clearly proposed to study and clarify the pharmacological effects of traditional Chinese medicine from the theory of traditional Chinese medicine.

TCM theory has its obvious overall view, emphasizing the balance of the body and maintaining balance when the internal and external environment changes. Losing balance and coordination, the body will have a medical certificate or a medical symptom.

Modern medicine also emphasizes the stability of the internal environment. The regulatory factors for the stability of the internal environment are the three systems of nerve, endocrine and immunity. These are self-contained systems that independently exert their respective regulatory roles, while at the same time interacting with each other and interacting with each other to achieve the goal of maintaining a relatively stable internal environment. **"Nerve and endocrine and immune regulatory networks" (NIM network) is currently a research hotspot in immunopharmacology. Professor Zhou Jin developed the NIM idea through a lot of research work, and believed that the "NIM" concept has broad practical significance**, is in line with the laws of life science, and coincides with the overall ideology of traditional Chinese medicine. Extensive and in-depth study of the role of traditional Chinese medicine in the NIM network can greatly develop the basic theories of Chinese medicine, so that Chinese medicine can go global faster.

Molecular level Chinese medicine research

---

13. The New finding from the experimental tumor research:

(1) Excision of the thymus (Thymus, TH) can be used to create a model of the animal model;

(2) The experimental results suggest that metastasis is related to immunity, and low immune function may promote tumor metastasis;

(3) The experimental results showed that the host thymus was acute progressive atrophy after inoculation of cancer cells, cell proliferation was blocked, and the volume was significantly reduced;

(4) The experimental results showed that when the transplanted solid tumor of the experimental mouse was long to the thumb, it was removed. After one week, the thymus was found to have no atrophy;

(5) Our laboratory is investigating the atrophy of the thymus gland in the immune organ to suppress the progression of the tumor, and looking for the method of immune reconstitution. The experimental study on the immune function of fetal liver, fetal thymus gland and fetal spleen cell transplantation was performed. The results showed that the three groups of S, T, L cells were transplanted. The complete regression rate of tumors was 40%, and the complete regression rate of long-term tumors was 46.67%.

From the above experimental studies, it is found that thymus atrophy and immune dysfunction may be one of the pathogenesis factors and pathogenesis of tumors. We should take the immune function from the body, especially cellular immunity, T lymphocyte function and thymus immune regulation function in the molecule. Explore the level and seek ways to regulate immune.

In view of the development of traditional Chinese medicine immunopharmacology, TCM theory has its obvious overall view, emphasizing the balance of the body, maintaining balance when the internal and external environment changes, losing balance, and the body has symptoms.

Modern medicine also emphasizes the stability of the internal environment and the regulation of the stable environment in the body. The factors are the three systems of nerve, endocrine and immunity. "Nerve, endocrine, and immunoregulatory networks" (NIM network) is currently a research hotspot in immunopharmacology.

Traditional Chinese medicine has a large number of prescriptions to regulate the body's immune function, especially the beneficial Chinese medicine has the effect of regulating immune activity. **In the past 60 years, we have conducted a series of experimental studies to find new anticancer drugs for anticancer, anticancer metastasis, prevention of thymic atrophy, and elevated immunity from natural drugs, and to find new anticancer drugs from natural** drugs; Look for drugs that are anti-metastatic and anti-relapse; look for drugs that only inhibit cancer cells without inhibiting normal cells; look for drugs that prevent thymic atrophy, regulate the regulation of host and tumor, and prevent recurrence and metastasis.

The existing anticancer drugs inhibit the immune function of the patient, inhibit the hematopoietic function of the bone marrow, inhibit the thymus, inhibit the bone marrow, and make it lose immune surveillance, so that the cancer can be further developed. Therefore, it is necessary to strengthen research so that all anticancer drugs used must be drugs that can boost immunity and protect immune organs, and should not be immune.

14. Study on the mechanism of XZ-C immunoregulation of anticancer traditional Chinese medicine

Looking for anti-cancer, anti-metastatic drugs within natural medicine (Chinese medicine):

In the experimental work, our laboratory has carried out long-term and batch-by-batch experiments on the anti-tumor screening of tumor-bearing animals in 200 traditional Chinese medicines that are considered to be "anti-cancer Chinese medicines". It was found that only 48 of them had certain or even better inhibitory effects on the proliferation of tumor cells. After optimized combination, the tumor-inhibiting experiment in tumor-bearing animal models such as liver cancer, lung cancer and gastric cancer is carried out.

Z-C1~10 particles are formed, Z-C1 can significantly inhibit cancer cells, but it does not affect normal cells. Z-C4 can protect the Thymus and improve immune function. Z-C8 can protect the marrow from blood. Z-C immunomodulatory Chinese medicine can improve the quality of life of patients with advanced cancer, increase immunity, enhance physical fitness, increase appetite and prolong survival.

With the deepening of research on traditional Chinese medicine, many traditional Chinese medicines are known to regulate the production and biological activities of cytokines and other immune molecules, which is of great significance for elucidating the immunological mechanism of Z-C immunomodulation of anticancer Chinese medicine at the molecular level.

(1) **XZ-C anti-cancer Chinese medicine can protect immune organs and increase the weight of thymus and spleen**

The role of XZ-C in protecting immune organs is exerted by the following active ingredients in the drug:

1. XZ-C-T (ASD)

Daily use of its extract (1g per liter of the original drug) 15g / kg, 30g / kg ferulic acid suspension 12.5mg / kg, 25mg / kg for mice, for 7d, can **significantly increase small Rat**

thymus and spleen weight, especially in the high dose group the effect is more obvious. Intraperitoneal injection of the polysaccharide into the mouse can also significantly reduce the atrophy of the thymus and spleen caused by prednisolone.

2. XZ-C-0 (PMT)

The extract PM-2 was given normal mice with PMT 6g/(kg•d) decoction for 7 days, which increased the weight of thymus and abdominal lymph nodes in mice. It can also antagonize the weight loss of immune organs caused by prednisolone. The 15-month-old mice were given 6 μg/kg of water decoction (concentration: 0.5 g/ml) for 14 days, which increased the weight and volume of the thymus in the mice, significantly thickened the cortex, and significantly increased the cell density.

The combination of PM and Astragalus can significantly promote non-lymphocyte proliferation and improve the thymus microenvironment.

3. XZ-C-W (SCB)

The polysaccharide of SCB can increase the weight of thymus and spleen in normal mice. It can also increase the weight of the thymus and spleen of cyclophosphamide immunosuppressed mice by gavage.

4. XZ-C-M (LLA)

When the mice were given LIA decoction for 7 days, the thymus and spleen weight index of the mice increased significantly.

5. XZ-C-L

The thymus of the mice at 15 months of age was significantly degraded, and the spleen was significantly increased by Astragalus injection. The light cortex was significantly thickened and the cell density was significantly increased under light microscope.

(2) **Effects of Z-C anticancer Chinese medicine on proliferation, differentiation and hematopoietic function of bone marrow cells**

The following active ingredients of Z-C Chinese medicine have an effect on the hematopoietic function of bone marrow.

The following active ingredients of Z-C Chinese medicine have an effect on the hematopoietic function of bone marrow.

1. Effects of Z-C-Q (PMT) extract (PM-2) and Z-C-Q (LBP) on normal mouse bone marrow hematopoietic stem cell proliferation (CFU-S):

The mice were intravenously injected with PM-2 at a dose of 50 mg/(kg•d)×3d or LBP at a dose of 10 mg/(kg•d)×3 days. The mice were killed on the 9th day. It was found that the number of spleen CFU-S in the mice in the drug-administered group increased significantly, and the CFU-S in the PM-2 group and the LBP group were 121% and 136% of the control group, respectively.

It can be seen from the above experiments that PM-2 and LBP have significant promoting effects on hematopoietic function in normal mice. The experiment proves: in the recovery process of hematopoietic damage induced by cyclophosphamide in mice, PM-2 and LBP first stimulated the proliferation of granulocyte progenitor cells, and then the nucleated cells of the bone marrow increased, and finally showed the recovery of peripheral granulocyte count.

2. XZ-C-D (TSPG):

Ginsenoside, which is the active principle of ginseng to promote hematopiesis, can bring the recovery of erythrocyte in peripheral blood, haemoglobin and myeloid cell of thighbone in the mice of marrow-inhibited type, increase the index of myeloid cellular division and stimulate the proliferation of myeloid hematopoietic cell in vitro so as to make it into cell cycle with active proliferation (S+G_2/M stage). TSPG can promote the proliferation and differentiation of polyenergetic hematopoietic cells and induce the formation of hemopoietic growth factor (HGF).

3. XZ-C-H (RCL):

Steamed Chinese Foxglove can promote the recovery of erythrocyte and haemoglobin for animals with blood deficiency and accelerate the proliferation and differentiation of myeloid hematopoietic cell (CFU-S) with the effect of predominance and hematosis significantly. Peritoneal injection of rehmannia polysaccharides for successive six days can promote the proliferation and differentiation of myeloid hematopoietic cells and progenitor cells as well as increasing the number of leucocytes in peripheral blood.

4. XZ-C-J (ASD):

ASD polysaccharide has no effects on erythrocytes and leucocytes of normal mice, but for those damaged by radiation, injection of ASD polysaccharide can influence the proliferation and differentiation of both polyenergetic hematopoietic stem cells (CPU-S) and hemopoietic progenitor cells. But its decoction has no obvious effects.

5. XZ-C-E (PEW):

Poria cocos (micromolecule chemical compound extracted from Tuckahoe polysaccharide) is the active principle that can strengthen the production of colony stimulating factor (CSF) and improve the level of leucocytes in peripheral blood inside the mouse's body. It can also prevent the decline in leucocytes caused by cyclophosphamide and accelerate the recovery with the effects better than sodium ferulic which is used to increase leucocytes.

6. XZ-C-Y (PAR):

Its polysaccharide can obviously resist the decline in leucocytes caused by cyclophosphamide and increase the number of myeloid cells to promote the proliferation of myeloid induced by CSF as well as the recovery and reconstitution of hematopiesis for the mice irradiated by X ray. It can also increase the number of hematopoietic stem cells and myeloid cells along with leucocytes.

(3) Enhancing Immunologic Function of T Cells

The active principles of XZ-C traditional Chinese medicine and their effects are following.

1. XZ-C-L (AMB): It can raise the percentage of lymphocytes in peripheral blood obviously. The LBP in small dose (5~10mg/kg) can cause the proliferation of lymphocytes, indicating that LBP can promote the proliferation of T cells apparently. 50mg/(kg·d)×7d is the best dose in that it will have no effects if lower than the level and it will bring the effects down if higher than the level. Oral administration of LBP can raise the conversion rate of lymphocytes for the sufferers who are weak and with fewer leucocytes.

2. XZ-C$_4$: It can regulate immune system and active T cells of aggregated lymphatic follicles, as well as stimulate the secretion of hemopoietic growth factor in T cells. Among the crude drugs of XZ-C$_4$, the extract from the hot water of atractylodes lancea rhizome can obviously stimulate the cells of aggregated lymphatic follicles, which is regarded as the base of XZ-C$_4$ immunoloregulation.

(4) Activating and Enhancing NK Cell Activity By XZ-C anticancer medications

Natural killer cell, NK cell is another kind of killer cell in lymphocytes for human beings and mice, which needs neither antigenic stimulation, nor the participation of antibodies to kill some cells. It plays an important role in immunity, especially in the function of immune surveillance as NK cell is the first line of defense against tumors and has broad spectrum anti-tumor effects.

NK cell is broad-spectrum and able to kill sygeneous, homogenous and heterogenous tumor cells with special effects on lymjphoma and leucocytes.

NK cell is an important kind of cells for immunoloregulation, which can regulate T cells, B cells and stem cells, etc. It can also regulate immunity by releasing cytokines like IFN-α, IFN-γ, IL-2, TNF, etc.

The active principles in XZ-C traditional Chinese medicine and their effects are following.

1. XZ-C-X (SDS)

Divaricate Saposhniovia Root can strengthen the activity of NK cells of experimental mice. When combined with IL-2, it can make the activity of NK cell higher, indicating that its polysaccharide can give a hand to IL-2 to activate NK cells and improve the activity.

LBP can strengthen T cell mediated immune reaction and the activity of NK cells for normal mice and those dealt by cyclophosphamide. Peritoneal injection of LBP can improve the proliferation of spleen T lymphocytes and strengthen the lethality of CTL increasing the specific lethal rate from 33% to 67%.

2. XZ-C-G (GUF)

Glycyrrhizin can induce the production of IFN in the blood of animals and human beings and strengthen NK cell activity at the same time. Clinical tests made by Abe show that after intravenous injection of 80mg GL, the raise of NK cell activity reaches 75% among 21 sufferers. Peritoneal injection of 0.5mg/kg GL on mice can strengthen the activity of NK cells in liver.

3. XZ-C-L (AMB)

Its bath fluid can promote NK cell activity of mice both in vivo and in vitro, and can also induce IFN-γ to deal with effector cells under the certain concentration of 0.1mg/ml. Cordyceps sinensis extract can strengthen NK cells activity of the mouse both in vivo and in vitro. Fluids with the concentrations of 0.5g/kg, 1g/kg and 5g/kg can strengthen NK cell activity of mice.

(5) Effects of ZX-C anti-cancer Chinese medications on Iterleukin-2 (IL-2)

The active principles in XZ-C anti-carcinoma traditional Chinese medicine and their effects are following.

1. XZ-C-T

EBM polysaccharide can enhance obviously the production of IL-2 for human beings when the concentration is 100ug/ml. At higher concentration (2500ug/ml and 5000ug/ml), it will lead to inhibition. Hypodermic injection of barrenwort polysaccharide for seven days in a row can significantly improve the ability of thymus and spleen of the mouse induced by ConA to produce IL-2.

2. XZ-C-Y

PAR polysaccharide has strong immune activity and is able to promote the production of IL-2. For the mouse bearing S-180 tumor, it can raise the ability of spleen cells to produce IL-2 obviously。

3. XZ-C-D

Ginseng polysaccharide has great promotion on IL-2 induced by peripheral monocytes for both healthy people and sufferers with kidney troubles. The effects are relevant to the dose positively.

IFN are broad-spectrum in resisting tumors and can regulate immunity. It can also inhibit the proliferation of tumor cells and activate NK cells and CTL to kill tumor cells. Meanwhile, IFN can cooperate with TNF, IL-1 and IL-2 to enforce anti-tumorous ability.

The active principles in XZ-C anti-carcinoma traditional Chinese medicine and their effects are following.

1. XZ-C-Z

250mg/kg or 500mg/kg CVQ polysaccharide can improve significantly the level of IFN-γ produced by mouse spleen cells.

2. XZ-C-D

Ginsenoside (GS) and panaxitriol ginsenoside (PTGS) can induce whole blood cells and monocytes of human beings to produce IFN-α and IFN-γ. It can also recover the low level of IFN-γ and IL-2 to the normal.

The IFN potency of ASH polysaccharide on S-180 cell line of acute lymphoblastic leukemia and S_{7811} cell line of acute myelomonocytic leukemia produced after acanthopanax polysaccharide stimulation is 5~10 times more than that of normal control group.

3. XZ-C-E

Hydroxymethyl Poria cocos mushroom polysaccharide has many kinds of physical activity like immunoloregulation, promoting to induce IPN, resisting virus indirectly and alleviating adverse reaction resulting from radiation. Do IFN inducement dynamic experiment on S-180leukaemia cell line by using 50mg/ml Hydroxymethyl Poria cocos mushroom polysaccharide. The results indicate that its potency to induce interferon at all stages is better than that of normal inducement.

4. XZ-C-G (GL)

It can induce IFN activity. Make peritoneal injection of 330mg/kg GL on mice. IFN activity reaches the peak after 20 hours.

15. The research of cytokines which are induced by XZ-C4 anticancer Chinese medications

(1) Z-C4 anticancer medications can induce endogenous cytokines

① The experimental study: Z-C4 has a variety of immune-enhancing effect and there are closely relation with induced endogenous cytokine.

② Z-C4 can inhibit the reduction of leukocyte and neutrophils and thrombocyte.

③ Through the interleukin -1β (IL-1β) Z-C4 not only has a direct effect on the production of GM-CSF, but also can enhance the tumor necrosis factor (TNF), interferon (IFN) and other cytokines, which may be an indirect mechanism.

④ In the cancer patients Th1 cytokine which regulates the cellular immune function decreases; however Z-C4 can raise Th1 cytokines so that it has effects on anemia and leukopenia after chemotherapy.

⑤ Z-C4 can not only protect the bone marrow, but also play a direct role in the cell differentiation through the cytokines.

In short, Z-C4 induces tumor cell differentiation and natural death due to autocrine which produce the different kind of cytokines. Autocrine is called as that the substance which is secreted by itself reversely acts on it own. Looking to the future, Z-C4 may become inducing therapy for cancer cell differentiation.

(2) Z-C4 can inhibit cancer progression and metastasis

Cancer cells obtains Invasion and metastasis of malignant nature in the proliferation process, this phenomenon is called malignant progression. To research cancer progress requires the good reproducibility animal model. Thus, the regression type of cancer cell QR-32 isolated from mouse fibrosarcoma was made into this good reproducibility animal model. Even though QR-32 was implanted subcutaneously in the mice, it was nor hyperplasia and will be completely self-limiting; it does not appear the metastatic nodules in the lung while it was injected through the vien. However, if the gelatin sponge as the foreign substances together with QR-32 was transplanted into mice subcutaneously, QR-32 becomes the proliferative cancer cell QRSP in vivo.

(3) Z-C1+Z-C4 immunomodulation anticancer Chinese medicine

Z-C1+Z-C4 immunomodulatory anticancer Chinese medicine has the following characteristics:

1. comprehensively improve the quality of life of patients with advanced cancer.
2. protect the thymus to improve immunity, protect the bone marrow, enhance hematopoietic function, improve immunity and regulation.

3. enhance physical fitness, reduce pain and increase appetite.
4. enhances the therapeutic effect and reduces the side effects of chemotherapy (Figures, the below).

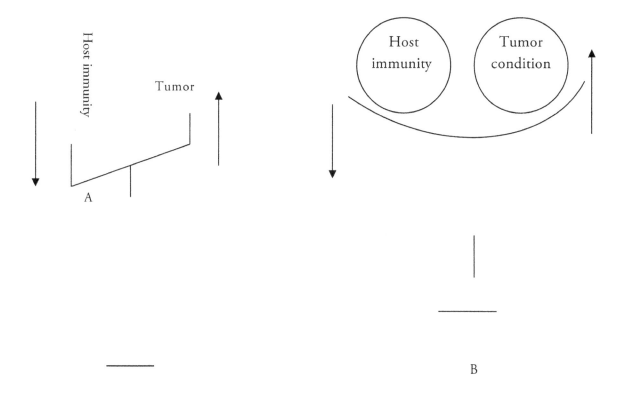

Fig. Schematics of "seesaw" and "weighing scale"

A. tumor grows up in unbalance; B. stabled improvement conditions in balance

16. The experiment and clinical efficacy of XZ-C immunomodulation anticancer Chinese medication

(1) **Antitumor effect of XZ-C$_1$ and XZ-C$_4$ anticancer Chinese medications on liver cancer in H$_{22}$ tumor-bearing mice**

It was found that after administrating the medications for 2 weeks, 4 weeks, and 6 weeks in the H$_{22}$ tumor-bearing mice, the tumor inhibition rate was increased with the prolonged medication administration time. The tumor inhibition rate of Z-C$_4$ at the 6th week was as high as 70%. After repeated tests twice, the results were stable, indicating that the anti-tumor effect of Chinese medicine is slow and gradually increased. That is, the anti-tumor effect is positively correlated with the cumulative dose of traditional Chinese medicine.

The effect of $Z\text{-}C_1$ and $Z\text{-}C_4$ anticancer Chinese medicine on the survival of H22 tumor-bearing mice:

The experimental results show that Z-C1, Z-C4 anti-cancer traditional Chinese medicine can significantly prolong the survival of tumor-bearing mice, especially Z-C4, significantly prolonging its survival time by more than 200%. Not only that, Z-C4 can significantly improve the body Immune function, protect immune organs, protect bone marrow, reduce the side effects of chemotherapy and radiotherapy drugs, and it has not seen any side effects after being fed for 12 months. The above experimental research provides a useful basis for clinical application.

(2) **Clinical efficacy**

On the basis of experimental research, since 1994, it has been applied to clinical cancers, mostly patients with stage III or IV. That is:

1). The advanced cancer that cannot be removed by exploration; 2). The advanced cancer has lost the indication for surgery; 3) recent or long-term metastasis or recurrence after various cancer operations;

4) liver metastasis, lung metastasis, brain metastasis or cancerous pleural effusion or cancerous ascites in various advanced cancers; 5) Various cancer with estimated resection, gastrointestinal anastomosis or colostomy can only be done but cannot be removed during the exploration; 6) Patients who are not suitable for surgery, radiotherapy or chemotherapy.

XZ-C1, XZ-C4 anti-cancer Chinese medicine has been clinically applied for 20 years, systematically observed, and achieved obvious curative effect. There are no side effects for long-term use. Clinical observations have shown that XZ-C1 andX Z-C4 anti-cancer traditional Chinese medications can comprehensively improve the quality of life of patients with advanced cancer, improve overall immunity, control cancer cell proliferation, and consolidate and enhance long-term efficacy. The internal and external application of XZ-C drug has a good effect on softening and reducing the surface metastasis of the tumor. Combined with intervention or intubation pump treatment, it can protect the liver, kidney, bone marrow hematopoietic system and immune organs and improve immunity.

(3) **The analgesic effect of XZ-C anti-cancer is good**

Pain in advanced cancer patients is more obvious and painful symptoms; the general pain medication does not have much effect for cancer pain and the narcotic analgesics are addiction and dependence; XZ-C anticancer analgesic cream has strong analgesic effect and last longer. In 298 cases it was clinically proved to have significantly effective rate 78.0%, the total efficiency of 95.3%, can be re-used with no significant side effects, non-addictive. Analgesic effect is stable and relieves pain for cancer patients to improve the quality of life.

Through experimental research and clinical validation, our experience is:

Traditional Chinese medicine with Chinese characteristics has its unique advantages in cancer treatment such as: Strong overall concept, the regulation effect is outstanding, mild side effects, alleviating the pain, relieving symptoms, significantly improving the quality of life of patients, and it can regulate the immune function of the body and the overall disease resistance and improving the treatment effect.

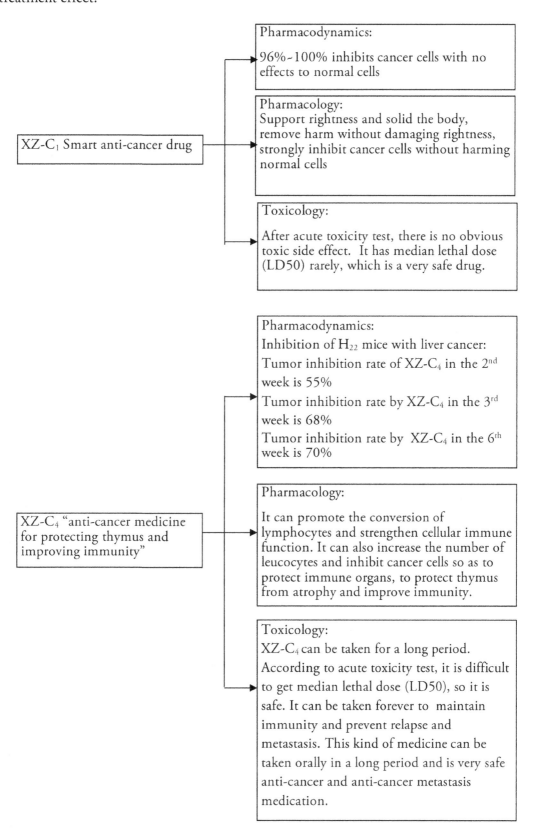

17. XZ-C immunomodulation anticancer Chinese medicine is the result of the modernization of traditional Chinese medicine

Exclusive research and development products:
A series of Z-C immune regulation anti-cancer Chinese medicine products (introduction)

The self-developed XZ-C (Xu Ze China) immune regulation and control anti-cancer series of traditional Chinese medicine preparations, from experimental research to clinical verification, applied to clinical practice on the basis of successful animal experiments, clinical practice of a large number of clinical cases over the years Verification, the effect is significant. For the independent invention results, it is independent innovation and independent intellectual property rights.

To search for and screen new anti-cancer and anti-metastatic drugs from traditional Chinese medicine:

The purpose is to screen out new anti-cancer, anti-metastatic, anti-recurrent and anti-cancer drugs that have no drug resistance, no toxic side effects, and high selectivity.

To this end, our laboratory conducted the following experimental studies to screen new anticancer and anti-metastatic drugs from traditional Chinese medicine:

(1) **Using the method of in vitro culture of cancer cells to conduct screening experiments on the rate of cancer suppression of Chinese herbal medicines:**

In vitro screening test: The cancer cells were cultured in vitro to observe the direct damage of the drug to cancer cells.

In-tube screening test: In the test tube for culturing cancer cells, the raw crude drug (500 ug/ml) was separately placed to observe whether it inhibited the cancer cells. We used 200 kinds of Chinese herbal medicines that traditional Chinese medicine believed to have anti-cancer effects. Screening experiments were performed in vitro. The toxicity of the drug to the cells was tested by normal fiber cell culture under the same conditions and then compared.

(2) **Making animal models of cancer-bearing animals, and conducting experimental screening of Chinese herbal medicines on the rate of cancer suppression in cancer-bearing animals**

In vivo anti-cancer screening test, 240 mice per batch were divided into 8 groups, 30 in each group, the 7th group was the blank control group, the 8th group was treated with 5-F or CTX as the control group, and the whole group was vaccinated with EAC or S180 or H22 cancer cells. After inoculation for 24 hours, each rat was orally fed with crude biological powder, and the selected traditional Chinese medicine was screened for a long time. The survival time, toxicity and side effects were observed, the survival rate was calculated, and the cancer inhibition rate was calculated

Therefore, we conducted experimental studies for four consecutive years in more than 1000 rats each year. A total of nearly 6,000 tumor-bearing animal models were made and autopsy each mice after died to observe liver, spleen, sheets, pituitary gland, kidney and to get pathological anatomy with a total of 20,000 slices to explore to find out whether There may be slight carcinogenic pathogens and the establishment of tumor micro-vessels beds and microcirculation was observed with the microscope in 100 tumor-bearing mice.

Through experimental study we first found that Chinese medication TG had a significant effect on inhibiting tumor angiogenesis. Now it has been used as anti metastasis in more than hundreds of the patients in clinic treatment.

Experimental results: In our laboratory animal experiments after screening 200 kinds of Chinese herbal medications, 48 kinds of medications with certain and excellent inhibitory effect on cancer cells and inhibition rate of more than 75-90% were selected. 152 kinds with no significant anti-cancer effects were screened-out.

48 kinds of traditional Chinese medications with having good tumor suppression rates after screening out were optimized into the combination and repeated tumor suppression rate experiments in vivo, and finally developed XU ZE China1-10(XZ-C1-10) immunomodulatory anticancer Chinese medication with Chinese characteristics.

$Z-C_1$ could inhibit cancer cells, but does not affect normal cells; $Z-C_4$ specially can increase thymus function, can promote proliferation, increased immunity; $Z-C_1$ can protect bone marrow function and to product more blood.

Clinical validation: Based on the success of animal experiments, clinical validation was conducted. Namely the oncology clinics and the Research Group of combined Chinese with Western medicine for anti-cancer and anti-metastasis and recurrence were established. The patient medical records were retained and the regular follow-up observation system were established to observe the long-term effects. From experimental research to clinical evidence, the new questions were discovered during the new clinical validation process, then went back to the laboratory for the basic research, then applied the results of a new experiment for clinical validation. Thus, the experiment to the clinics, the experiment again and the clinical experiment again, all experimental studies must be clinically proven in a large number of patients observed 3--5 years, or even clinical observation of 8 to 10 years. According to evidence-based medicine, the long-term follow-up assessment information had gained and they have been verified indeed to have a good long-term efficacy. The efficacy of the standard is: a good quality of life, longer survival. XZ-C sectional immune regulation anti-cancer medicine was made after a lot of applications in advanced cancer patients verification and achieved remarkable results and can improve the quality of life of patients with advanced cancer, enhance immune function, increase the body's anticancer abilities, increased appetite and significantly prolong survival.

Many of Chinese herbal medicines are immune enhancers, biological response modifiers, and tonics, many of which can strengthen the body's immunity and anti-cancer power. The two world diseases that currently threaten human life are cancer and AIDS. **The former is immunocompromised and the latter is immunodeficient**. At present, scientists all over the world agree that tumor formation is summarized into three processes: the first step is that carcinogenic factors act on the body and interfere with cell metabolism; the second step is to disrupt the genetic information in the nucleus and cause cell cancer; the third step is that cancer cells escape the body. The immune alert defense system, the body's immune defense ability is an internal cause, and the external cause works through internal factors. Cancer cells must be able to escape the monitoring system of the body's alarm system, breaking through the body's immune defense line, in order to develop into a tumor. Therefore, trying to improve the body's immunity is the key measure to prevent cancer and cancer. How to improve immunity? Chinese herbal medicine is an extremely important advantage. There are many immune Chinese herbal preparations, which are rich in medicine sources. It should be used as an important preventing cancer and anti-cancer resource for tissue research and development. The research of the prevention and treatment of malignant tumors in the world are carried out in each country. Each country focuses on a large number of experts and scholars with the experimental research and clinical experience to study and try to overcome cancer.

We should be in the advantage areas in our country to play the advantages of our country and to catch up with the international advanced level.

In the field of cancer research, the traditional Chinese medication is the advantage of our country. To play this advantage in the function of the field of cancer research and to explore and to develop the prevention of the cancer and anti - cancer Chinese herbal medications and to play this advantage of the study should be a strategic significance of the international significance.

On the road of human conquest cancer the research and the excavation and the development of effective and reproducible anti-cancer anti-cancer new Chinese herbal medication preparations must be promising and can be excavated into effective treasure and must be carried out the strict and objective and realistic and scientific and repetitive research with the strict scientific methods and the modern experimental surgical methods. All experimental studies must be rigorously and clinically proven in a large number of patients who demonstrate that there is a good curative effect and that the standard of efficacy is good quality of life and prolonged survival.

A series of products of XZ-C immunoregulation anti-cancer traditional Chinese medicine

1. **XZ-C1+4: for all kinds of cancer**
2. **XZ-C1: has the stable and significant anti-cancer effects, the inhibition rate up to 98%, no harmful to normal cells.**
3. **XZ-C4: protection of thymus and increase of immune function, promote the thymus proliferation, increase the immune function**

   XZ-C8: protection of bone marrow and production of blood, increase T cells, and anti-metastasis

4. **Lung cancer: XZ-C1+XZ-C4+XZ-C7**
5. **Breast cancer: XZ-C+XZ-C+XZ-C+ mushroom**
6. **Esphogus cancer: XZ-C1+XZ-C4+XZ-C2**
7. **Stomach cancer: XZ-C1+XZ-C4 or +XZ-C5**
8. **Liver Ca: XZ-C1+XZ-C4+XZ-C5 + Mushroom+ Red ginseng**
9. **Bile cancer: XZ-C1+XZ-C4+XZ-C5 + Capillaris**
10. **Pancrease cancer: XZ-C1+XZ-C4+XZ-C5+XZ-C9**
11. **Colon and rectal cancer: XZ-C1+XZ-C4+XZ-C5**
12. **Kidney and bladder cancer: XZ-C1+XZ-C4+XZ-C6**
13. **Cervical and ovary cancer: XZ-C1+XZ-C4+XZ-C5+ Lms+ MDS**
14. **Lymphma: XZ-C1+XZ-C4+XZ-C2+ Dai Dai**
15. **Leukemia: XZ-C1+XZ-C4+XZ-C2+XZ-C8+ barge pole**
16. **Prostate cancer:XZ-C1+XZ-C4+XZ-C6**

Comments: *A series of XZ-C immune regulation anti-cancer traditional medications have been verified and tested for 20 years in Shuguang tumor special out-patient center on 12,000 of middle or later stage cancer patients. On clinical application they can change the symptoms, the patients have the good spirit and appetites are good, thlife quality is improved, and they significantly prolong the survival time.*

Adaptation Scope of Clinical application observation of XZ-C immunomodulation Chinese medication XZ-C$_{1-10}$ anti-cancer metastasis and recurrence

1. a variety of distant metastatic cancer, such as liver metastases, lung metastases, bone metastases, brain metastases, abdominal lymph node metastasis, mediastinal lymph node metastasis, cancerous pleural effusion, cancerous ascites, can be applied XZ-C immunization Regulate and Control anti-metastatic treatment, according to the transfer step, intervene and block the cancer cells on the way to prolong life.

2. After all kinds of radiotherapy and chemotherapy have been completed, XZ-C1-4 should be taken to control the traditional Chinese medicine to consolidate the long-term effect and prevent recurrence.

3. in the process of radiotherapy and chemotherapy, if the reaction is serious and can not continue, you can continue to use XZ-C immunomodulation therapy to resist metastasis and recurrence.

4. in the elderly or weak patient with other diseases who cannot have radiology and chemotherapy, XZ-C immunomodulation anti-metastasis, relapse treatment.

5. surgical exploration can not be cut, can be used XZ-C immune regulation treatment.

6. after palliative surgery, XZ-C immunomodulation anti-metastatic treatment.

7. after a variety of cancer radical surgery, should continue to take XZ-C immunomodulation treatment of traditional Chinese medicine anti-recurrence, metastasis, in order to improve the long-term effect after radical surgery

Second, the Guidance or introduction - "finding the road"

Walked out the new road to conquer cancer in the past more than 60 years

Research inspiration from walked out a new road - pathfinding

Conquer cancer, where is the direction of the road? - Where is the road? Where to go? How to find this way?

What new road did we walk on in cancer treatment?

We have been walking on and are taking a new road combining Chinese and Western medicine; it is a new way of combining Chinese and Western medicine at the molecular level; it is a new way for our laboratory to find immunomodulatory methods and drugs based on the new findings of animal experiments; after years of animal experiment screening And clinical verification, finally looking for a new way of immunomodulation with XZ-C immune regulation and control anti-cancer Chinese medicine series.

Why should we take a new road combining Chinese and Western medicine? Why should we take a new path of combining Western medicine at the molecular level? Why should we take a new path to find immunomodulatory drugs?

The road we are looking for is a step-by-step process that has gone through more than 20 years of clinical validation. It is not at the beginning having this understanding; Instead, I gradually realized it step by step.

Cancer treatment innovation road

We are taking the new road of "Chinese-style anti-cancer" combining Chinese and Western medicine and combining Western medicine with anti-cancer at the molecular level.

The combination of Chinese and Western medicine is the characteristics and advantages of Chinese medicine. The goal of combining Chinese and Western medicine should be to combine innovation, and the goal of innovation should be to improve the treatment effect. The efficacy criteria for cancer patients should be: **long survival time, good quality of life, and few complications.**

In the past 60 years, we have initially embarked on a new way to use immunomodulation of Chinese medicine, regulate immune activity, prevent thymic atrophy, promote thymic hyperplasia, protect bone marrow hematopoietic function, improve immune surveillance, and combine Western medicine at the molecular level to overcome cancer.

Our experimental surgical research institute is based on the research of cancer and the main task, focusing on the major topic of conquering cancer, taking the road of combining Chinese and Western medicine, and conducting research on the combination of Chinese and Western medicine at the molecular level. On the basis of animal experiment research, And in the clinical practice to achieve the combination of Chinese and Western medicine, and then in the anti-cancer, anti-cancer transfer theory development, innovation:

Adhering to the scientific research work of combining Chinese and Western medicine with innovation, we should persevere and persevere, adhere to the road of independent innovation with Chinese characteristics, and promote the new development of the theory of modern oncology in the 21st century.

Efforts will be made to take the road of innovation in China's distinctive anti-cancer transfer, take the road of modernization of traditional Chinese medicine, promote the integration of Chinese and Western medicine at the molecular level, and integrate with international medicine modernization. We have embarked on a road of XZ-C immune regulation, molecular and Chinese medicine combined with cancer. - "Chinese-style anti-cancer" new road.

[Note]:

- *"Chinese-style anti-cancer" is a monograph title published by Academician Tang Yu in April 2014. The wisdom of Sun Tzu's art of war is used for anti-cancer strategy and tactical thinking.*
- *I think that the combination of Chinese and Western medicine is only a method, and it is a means. Why should we combine Chinese and Western medicine? How to combine Chinese and Western medicine? What is the goal of the combination? Academician Wu Xianzhong proposed that the goal of combining Chinese and Western medicine should be to combine innovation.*
- *So what is the goal of combining innovation? What are the hopes of combining innovation?*
- *I believe that the goal of combining innovation is to improve the effectiveness of treatment and benefit patients. The efficacy of cancer patients should be: long survival time, good quality of life, and fewer complications.*
- *The result of combining innovation should be innovation "Chinese medicine" innovation "Chinese-style anti-cancer".*

If this sentence is analyzed in a sentence, it should be:

Subject	Predicate	
Integrating Chinese and Western Medicine	combine to innovation	Innovating "Chinese Medicine" and Innovating "Chinese Anti-Cancer"
Subject(S)	(V) Verb	(O) Object

This is only a complete sentence, with purpose, method, and result, so I quote the word "Chinese-style anti-cancer" created by Academician Tang Yu. It is also the new way of combining the ideological understanding and research thinking of our scientific research journey that the anti-cancer and anti-metastatic research institutes have gone through in the past 60 years.

The theory of Cancer treatment innovation

Pathfinding – Looking for where the road is?

The road we have been looking for in the past 60 years has come over just like this step by step:

- Discovery of findings through follow-up:

(1) - Looking for ways to prevent and treat cancer after recurrence and metastasis
(method, medicine, technology, basic theory)

- Discovery through the findings of experimental research:

(2) - Looking for ways to prevent thymus atrophy, promote thymic hyperplasia, and boost immunity
(method, medicine, technology, basic theory)

(3) - Looking for the road to immune reconstruction
(method, medicine, technology, basic theory)

- Through our proposed anti-cancer metastasis research on the new concept of cancer metastasis, the new theory of understanding: the key to cancer treatment is anti-metastasis, how to eliminate the cancer cell group on the way to transfer.

(4) - Looking for ways to eliminate cancer cells on the way to metastasis
(method, medicine, technology, basic theory)

- Through the above research results: We basically found the way to take immunomodulatory therapy, and gradually established XZ-C immunomodulation therapy.

We think this is one of the roads to overcome cancer. In order to explore the etiology, pathogenesis and pathophysiology of cancer, we conducted a series of animal experiments. From the experimental results, we obtained new findings, new inspirations: thymus atrophy, and low immune function is one of the causes and pathogenesis of cancer. Therefore, Xu Ze (Xu Ze) proposed one of the causes and pathogenesis of cancer at international conferences, which may be thymus atrophy, central immune organ damage, immune dysfunction, decreased immune surveillance, and immune escape.

Regardless of the complexity of the mechanisms behind cancer, mechanismic immunosuppression is the key to cancer progression. Removing immunosuppressive factors and restoring the recognition of cancer cells by immune system cells may effectively prevent cancer.

By activating the body's anti-tumor immune system to treat tumors, a major breakthrough in the next cancer is likely to stem from this. Immunomodulatory therapy, the prospects are gratifying.

In 1985, I conducted a petition with more than 3,000 patients who underwent radical surgery for various cancers. It was found that most patients had recurrence and metastasis 2 to 3 years after surgery, and some even metastasized several months after surgery. This made me realize that although the operation is successful, the long-term efficacy is not satisfactory. Postoperative recurrence and metastasis are the key factors affecting the long-term efficacy of the operation. It also reminds us that prevention and treatment of postoperative recurrence and metastasis is the key to prolonging postoperative survival. Therefore, basic research must be carried out, and without breakthroughs in basic research, clinical efficacy is difficult to improve. So we established the Institute of Experimental Surgery and spent a total of 34 years conducting a series of experimental research and clinical validation work from the following three aspects.

1. Explore the mechanism of cancer onset, invasion and recurrence and metastasis, and carry out experimental research on effective measures to regulate invasion, recurrence and metastasis.

We have been conducting laboratory research for a full four years in the laboratory. They are clinical basic research and research projects. They are all clinically raised questions to explain these clinical problems or solve these clinical problems through experimental research.

From experimental tumor research it was found:

(1) Resection of the thymus (Thymus, TH) can produce a cancer-bearing animal model;
(2) The experimental results suggest that metastasis is related to immunity, and low immune function may promote tumor metastasis;
(3) The experimental results showed that the host thymus was acute progressive atrophy after inoculation of cancer cells, cell proliferation was blocked, and the volume was significantly reduced;
(4) The experimental results showed that when the transplanted solid tumor of the experimental mouse grew long or big to the thumb, it was removed. After one week, the thymus was found to have no atrophy;
(5) Our laboratory is investigating the atrophy of the thymus gland in the immune system to stop the progression of the tumor, and looking for the method of immune reconstitution. The experimental study on the immune function of fetal liver, fetal thymus gland and fetal spleen cell transplantation was used to reconstruct the immune function. The

results showed that the three groups of S, T, L cells were transplanted. The complete regression rate of tumors was 40%, and the complete regression rate of long-term tumors was 46.67%.

Our laboratory experimental results showed that the thymus of the cancer-bearing mice showed progressive atrophy, the volume was reduced, the cell proliferation was blocked, and the mature cells were reduced. By the end of the tumor, the thymus is extremely atrophied and the texture becomes hard.

From the above experimental studies, it is found that thymus atrophy and immune dysfunction may be one of the pathogenic factors and pathogenesis of tumors, so it is necessary to try to prevent thymus atrophy, promote thymocyte proliferation, and increase immunity. The immune function of the body, especially cellular immunity, the function of T lymphocytes, and the immune regulation function of the thymus should be explored at the molecular level, and methods for immune regulation and effective drug research should be sought.

It should further carry out the research from the thymus function and tissue structure, immune function is low and how to promote immunity, immune reconstitution, how to "protect the thymus and increase immune functions" and look for new ways and new methods of cancer treatment.

2. The experimental research of looking for new drug with anti-cancer, anti-metastatic, anti-recurrence from natural drugs.

The existing anticancer drugs kill both cancer cells and normal cells, and have large adverse reactions. We have tried new cancer drugs in cancer-bearing mice to find new drugs that inhibit cancer cells without affecting normal cells. We spent a full three years on the anti-tumor screening experiments of cancer-bearing animals in 200 kinds of Chinese herbal medicines used in traditional anti-cancer agents and anti-cancer agents reported in various places. Results 48 kinds of traditional Chinese medicines with good anti-tumor effect and good effects were screened out.

To search for and screen new anti-cancer and anti-metastatic drugs from traditional Chinese medicine:

The purpose is to screen out new anti-cancer, anti-metastatic, anti-recurrent and anti-cancer drugs that **have no drug resistance, no toxic side effects, and high selectivity.**

To this end, our laboratory conducted the following experimental studies to screen new anticancer and anti-metastatic drugs from traditional Chinese medicine:

(1)   Using the method of in vitro culture of cancer cells, screening experiments on the cancer suppression rate of Chinese herbal medicines:

In vitro screening test: The cancer cells were cultured in vitro to observe the direct damage of the drug to cancer cells.

In-vitro screening test, in the test tube for culturing cancer cells, respectively, into the crude drug product (500 ug / ml), to observe whether it has an inhibitory effect on cancer cells, we will take 200 kinds of Chinese herbal medicines that traditional Chinese medicine thinks have anti-cancer effect. Screening experiments were performed in vitro. The toxicity of the drug to the cells was tested by normal fiber cell culture under the same conditions and then compared.

(2)   Making animal models of cancer-bearing animals, and conducting experimental screening of Chinese herbal medicines on cancer suppression rate in cancer-bearing animals

In vivo anti-cancer screening test, each batch of 240 mice, divided into 8 groups, 30 in each group, the seventh group was a blank control group, the eighth group with 5-FU or CTX as a control group, the whole group of mice Inoculate EAC or S180 or H22 cancer cells. After inoculation for 24 hours, each rat was orally fed with crude drug powder, and the traditional Chinese medicine was screened for a long time. The survival time, toxicity and side effects were calculated, the survival rate was calculated, and the cancer inhibition rate was calculated.

In this way, we conducted a four-year experimental study, and conducted an experimental study on the pathogenesis, metastasis, and recurrence mechanism of tumor-bearing mice for three years, and an experimental study to explore how tumors cause host death. More than 1,000 tumor-bearing animals are used each year. In the model, nearly 6000 tumor-bearing animal models were made in 4 years. After the death of each mouse, the pathological anatomy of the liver, spleen, lung, thymus and kidney was performed. More than 20,000 slices were taken to explore whether to find out whether there may be carcinogenic micro-pathogens, and microcirculation microscopy was used to observe the microvascular establishment and microcirculation in the 100 tumor-bearing mice.

Through experimental research, we have found for the first time in China that TG has a significant effect on inhibiting tumor microvessel formation. It has been used in more than 80 clinical patients for anti-metastasis treatment.

Experimental results: Among the 200 kinds of Chinese herbal medicines screened by animal experiments in our laboratory, 48 kinds of selected and even excellent tumor cell proliferation were inhibited, and the tumor inhibition rate was above 75~90%. However, there are also some commonly used traditional Chinese medicines that are generally considered to have anti-cancer effects. After screening for animal tumors in vitro and in vivo, there is no anti-cancer effect, or the effect is very small. In this group, 152 kinds of anti-cancer effects were eliminated by animal experiments.

The 48 kinds of traditional Chinese medicines with good cancer suppression rate were selected by this experiment, and then the optimized combination was repeated to carry out the experiment of cancer suppression rate in cancer. Finally, the immune-regulating and controlling anti-cancer Chinese medicine XU ZE China$_{1-10}$ preparation (XZ-C$_{1-10}$) with its own characteristics was developed.

XZ-C1 can significantly inhibit cancer cells, but does not affect normal cells; XZ-C4 can promote thymic hyperplasia and increase immunity; XZ-C8 can protect the marrow from hematopoiesis and protect bone marrow hematopoietic function.

3. How should we find new ways to regulate immune therapy?

In order to try to prevent thymus atrophy, promote thymocyte proliferation, increase immunity, we look for both Chinese medicine and western medicine. The existing medicines of western medicine which can improve immunity and promote the proliferation of thymus is few. So we changed to look for Chinese herbal medicine.

(1) Why do you look for drugs that promote thymic hyperplasia, prevent thymus atrophy, and boost immunity? Because Chinese medicine's tonic drugs generally contain the role of regulating immunity.

1. Chinese medicine, polysaccharide Chinese medicine, tonic medicine, many of them have the role of regulating immunity.

The role of traditional Chinese medicine in regulating immune function is generally replenishing, and traditional Chinese medicine for tonic has the effect of regulating immune activity. Replenishing drugs can be called immunomodulatory drugs, causing non-specific immune responses.

Chinese medicines for tonics have the function of regulating the immune function of the body. Under the general experimental conditions, the correlation between dose and benefit is presented, especially in normal healthy animal experiments. When animals are at low levels of immune activity (such as dethymus, aging animals or chemotherapy drugs cyclophosphamide inhibition and tumor animals), the tonic drugs improve the body's immunity is more significant.

2. Research on anti-cancer immunity of Chinese medicine polysaccharides is progressing rapidly. A large number of immunopharmacological studies have been carried out at the molecular level. Polysaccharides can improve the body's immune surveillance system, including natural killer cells (NK), macrophages (MΦ), and killer T cells. (CTL), T cells, LAK cells, tumor infiltrating lymphocytes (TIL), interleukin (IL) and other cytokines are active to kill tumor cells. Although many polysaccharides have a certain anti-tumor effect, the two immunopotentiators, including the two polysaccharides, have a higher therapeutic effect.

Traditional Chinese medicine and western medicine have their own strengths, each with its own shortness. Compared with Western medicine immunopharmacology, traditional Chinese medicine immunopharmacology has its own characteristics or advantages, and each has its own shortcomings. The advantages of traditional Chinese medicine immunology are as follows:

A large number of Chinese medicines have the effect of regulating the body's immune function, especially the beneficial Chinese medicines generally have the effect of regulating immune activity.

Chinese medicine is rich in source and is an effective medicine for long-term clinical treatment. After extraction, it can obtain active ingredients and have obvious pharmacological effects (including immunomodulatory effects). The research process saves people time and has high efficiency.

(2) Why look for immunomodulatory drugs from traditional Chinese medicine, because of the progress in the study of traditional Chinese medicine immunopharmacology.

In view of the development of traditional Chinese medicine immunopharmacology, TCM theory has its obvious overall view, emphasizing the balance of the body, maintaining balance; when the internal and external environment changes and loses balance, the body has disease symptoms.

Modern medicine also emphasizes the stability of the internal environment and the regulation of the stable environment in the body. The factors are the three systems of nerve, endocrine and immunity. "Nerve, endocrine, and immunoregulatory networks" (NIM network) is currently a research hotspot in immunopharmacology.

Traditional Chinese medicine has a large number of prescriptions to regulate the body's immune function, especially the beneficial Chinese medicine has the effect of regulating immune activity. In the past 60 years, our laboratory has carried out a series of experimental studies to find new anticancer drugs for anticancer, anticancer metastasis, thymus atrophy, and immune enhancement from natural drugs, and to find new anticancer drugs from natural drugs. Looking for anti-metastatic, anti-relapsing drugs; looking for drugs that only inhibit cancer cells without inhibiting normal cells; looking for drugs that prevent thymic atrophy, regulate host-tumor regulation, and prevent recurrence and metastasis.

The existing chemotherapy anticancer drugs inhibit the immune function of the patient, inhibit the hematopoietic function of the bone marrow, inhibit the thymus, inhibit the bone marrow, and make it lose immune surveillance, so that the cancer can be further developed. Therefore, it is necessary to strengthen research so that all anticancer drugs used must be drugs that can boost immunity and protect immune organs, and should not be immune.

(3) Why did it look for drugs that promote thymic hyperplasia, prevent thymus atrophy, and boost immunity from traditional Chinese medicine? Because in the course of our research on anti-cancer and anti-cancer metastasis, we gradually discovered and recognized that the theory of traditional Chinese medicine is similar to our concept and principles of anti-cancer and anti-cancer metastasis, and even has some similarities.

Chinese medicine theory	New concept of anti-cancer and anti-cancer metastasis research
1、**a.** TCM treatment believes that righteousness is not Fictitious or imaginary, evil spirits do not enter, governance and treatment must be righteous and firm the solid and increase tonic. **b. And** developed a series of prescriptions for tonic drugs. The essence is to maintain the overall functional balance and enhance disease resistance. **c.** In modern scientific language, the main role of supplemental drugs is to enhance the body's immune function. **d.** In Chinese medicine treatment it is to emphasize righting and is equivalent to the immune function of Western medicine.	1、**a.** Our experimental study found that: tumor model has thymus atrophy, immune function is low, it must try to prevent thymus atrophy, promote thymocyte proliferation, increase immunity, it must seek to enhance immune drugs to enhance immunity. **b.** Therefore, the theory of traditional Chinese medicine is in good agreement with the concept of the new concept and new method of cancer metastasis. **c.** We understand the supporting rightness and solidification of traditional Chinese medicine, which is equivalent to the immunity of Western medicine and enhance the body's disease resistance.
2、**a.** TCM treatment not only pays attention to righting up, but also pays attention to evil spirits, that is, helping the righteousness and removing evils or strengthening the righteousness can kill the evil spirits. **b. The** traditional Chinese medicine rightness and removing evils are based on the treatment of increasing immune function in Western medicine, thereby improving the treatment principle of immune surveillance to eliminate metastasize cancer cells. The two are in good agreement。	2、**a.** The traditional concept of Western medicine believes that cancer is the continuous division and proliferation of cancer cells, and the goal of treatment must be to kill cancer cells. **b.** The new concept and new method of cancer metastasis we studied believe that the treatment and cure of cancer should be regulated and controlled rather than killed. **c.** Protecting the thymus and improving immunity and improving immune surveillance and controlling the transfer of cancer cells are similar to the concept of evil spirits in the Chinese medicine practitioners.

3、**a.** Traditional Chinese medicine treatment of activation of blood and removing stasis are a common treatment principle, so it is commonly used to promote blood circulation and to remove blood stasis drugs.

b. There are many drugs with circulating-blood and removing blood stasis in traditional Chinese medicine, the effect is exact, the effect is long-lasting, and it can be taken orally for a long time. It is suitable for anti-cancer metastasis drugs, because anti-cancer and anti-metastatic drugs must be taken orally for a long time.

c. Traditional Chinese medication has many medications with blood-activating circulation and removing the blood stasis, which can be used for anti-cancer thrombosis and prevention of cancer thrombosis and anti-cancer metastasis.

From the << new concept and new method of cancer metastasis treatmenth>> research it is believed that cancer cells in the blood circulation are gathered into a heap, surrounded by cellulose, platelets and a small amount of white blood cells to form tiny tumor thrombi. The tumor thrombus can be transported to other parts by blood flow, or stayed primary site after a certain period of time, it can penetrate the local upper wall, adhere to the solid organ cells and divide and proliferate around the blood vessel and forms the metastasis.

3、**a. From** the << new concept and new method of cancer metastasis treatmenth>> research it is believed that cancer cells in the blood circulation are gathered into a heap, surrounded by cellulose, platelets and a small amount of white blood cells to form tiny tumor thrombi. The tumor thrombus can be transported to other parts by blood flow, or stayed primary site after a certain period of time, it can penetrate the local upper wall, adhere to the solid organ cells and divide and proliferate around the blood vessel and forms the metastasis.

b. In our research on anti-cancer metastasis, we realized that we must focus on the cancer cell population or cancer cell groups or micro-cancer plugs on the metastasis way and conduct the encircling, chasing, blocking, intercepting, and anti-coagulation. Anti-coagulation is the main point of anti-cancer.

c. How to eliminate cancer cells and tumor thrombus on the way of metastasis?

4. Clinical verification work

(1)   After 7 years of scientific experiments in the laboratory, the XZ-C immunomodulatory anti-cancer and anti-metastatic traditional Chinese medicines with protection of Thymus and increase immune function and protection of bone marrow and production of blood and promote blood circulation and reduction of blood stasis. On the basis of the success of animal experiments, clinical validation work was carried out.

(2) Since 1985, one side is that the tumor-bearing mice in the tumor-bearing mice has been done, one side has been tested in clinical practice.

However, there are few patients, and there is no medical record in the outpatient clinic (the medical records are all issued to patients), and it is impossible to accumulate scientific research materials. It must take the road of scientific research and cooperation.

(3) Establishing an anti-cancer research collaboration group, taking the road of scientific research collaboration and joint research, and setting up the Dawn Cancer Specialist Clinic.

(4) Resume the outpatient medical records, fill in the complete and detailed outpatient medical records, obtain complete information of clinical verification, facilitate analysis and statistics, and be conducive to outpatient clinical research to improve the quality of medical care.

(5) Retaining outpatient cases, regular follow-up, and a brief analysis of the experience and lessons of this case, in order to long-term observation of long-term efficacy.

(6) The oncology clinic outpatient medical records are designed in a tabular format, including all relevant medical information and relevant epidemiological data, in order to statistically analyze the possible pathogenic factors.

(7) Cases and outpatient medical records that have been reviewed for more than 1 year, all of which are written with medical records, and analyzed on a large scale. The contents of the large table include the contents of the outpatient medical record form, which are both concise and detailed, and the Twilight Oncology Specialist The outpatient clinic has been verified for 35 years, and the large scale has accumulated nearly 10,000 outpatient clinical data for outpatient clinical research.

(8) From experimental research to clinical research, from clinical to experimental. The collaboration group has an experimental research base and a clinical application verification base. The former is in the medical laboratory, and the latter is in the Twilight Oncology Clinic. From the experiment to the clinical, that is, based on the success of the experimental research, it is applied to the clinical and clinical application process. New problems are discovered, and further basic experimental research is carried out, and new experimental results are applied to clinical verification. For example, outpatients have liver cancer with portal vein tumor thrombus, renal cancer patients with inferior vena cava tumor thrombus, some are CT reports, and some are surgery. The pathological section of the specimen was resected. **In fact, the cancerous tumor is the cancer cell group on the way to metastasis. It is the third manifestation of cancer in the human body. When the cancer thrombosis problem is discovered, we began the experimental study of cancer thrombus formation. Looking for new ways to fight against cancerous plugs and dissolve cancerous plugs, we found four traditional Chinese medicines that help to dissolve cancerous plugs and found out their active ingredients.**

Such experiments → clinical → re-experiment → re-clinical, continuous cyclical rise, after 12 years of clinical practice experience, understanding is also constantly rising, summed up practice, analysis, reflection, evaluation has risen to theory, propose new understanding, new thinking, new Treatment ideas.

(9) **Clinical efficacy observation:** On the basis of experimental research, it has been applied to clinical cancers since 1994, mostly patients with stage III or IV, ie advanced cancer that cannot be removed by exploration; recent cancer surgery Or long-term metastasis or recurrence; liver metastasis, lung metastasis, brain metastasis, bone metastasis or cancerous pleural effusion, cancerous ascites in various advanced cancers; palliative resection of various cancers, exploration can only do stomach Thoracic anastomosis or colostomy and can not be removed; patients who are not suitable for surgery, radiotherapy or chemotherapy. XZ-C immunomodulation anticancer Chinese medicine has been clinically applied for 34 years, and systematic observation has achieved obvious curative effect. No adverse reactions were observed after long-term use. Clinical observations have shown that XZ-C immunomodulatory Chinese medicine can comprehensively improve the quality of life of patients with advanced cancer, improve immunity, control cancer cell proliferation, and consolidate and enhance long-term efficacy after surgery or radiotherapy.

(10) Oral administration and external application of XZ-C medicine have good curative effect on softening and reducing surface metastasis of tumor. Combined with intervention or intubation pump treatment, it can protect liver, kidney, bone marrow hematopoietic system and immune organs and improve immunity.

In the Dawn Cancer Specialist Clinic, 4698 cases of stage III, IV or metastatic recurrent cancer were treated for long-term follow-up or follow-up.

(11) **Evaluation of quality of life of patients with advanced cancer by XZ-C immunomodulation Chinese medicine**: This group is middle and late stage patients, the symptom improvement rate is 93.2%, the mental improvement is 95.2%, the appetite is improved by 93%, and the physical strength is increased by 57.3. %, comprehensively improved the quality of life of patients with advanced cancer.

(12) Efficacy evaluation: not only pay attention to the short-term efficacy and imaging indicators, but also pay attention to the long-term efficacy of survival, quality of life and immune indicators, **the goal is to live long patients, good quality of life. During the course of medication,** it is necessary to pay attention to changes in symptoms and improvement of symptoms during medication; it is effective for lasting more than 1 month, otherwise it is invalid; it pays attention to the spirit, appetite, and quality of life (Carson's score).

From experimental research to clinical validation, new problems are discovered during the clinical validation process, and back to the laboratory for basic research, and new experimental results are applied to clinical validation. For example, experiment-clinical-re-experiment-re-clinical, all experimental research must be clinically verified. In a large number of patients, observe for 3 to 5 years, or even clinical observation for 8 to 10 years. According to evidence-based medicine, there is long-term prevention. The interview and evaluable data prove that there is a good long-term efficacy. The standard of efficacy is: good quality of life and long survival. XZ-C immunomodulation anticancer traditional Chinese medicine preparation has been proved to be effective after being applied to a large number of patients with advanced cancer. XZ-C immunomodulatory Chinese medicine can improve the quality of life of patients with advanced cancer, enhance immunity, enhance the body's ability to fight cancer, enhance appetite, and significantly prolong survival.

5. The mechanism of action of XZ-C immune regulation of anti-cancer Chinese medicine

XZ-C immunomodulatory Chinese medicine can improve the quality of life of patients with advanced cancer, enhance immunity, enhance the body's ability to fight cancer, enhance appetite, and significantly prolong survival. The introduction is as follows:

With the deepening of research on traditional Chinese medicine, many traditional Chinese medicines have been known to regulate the production and biological activities of cytokines and other immune molecules. At this time, the immunological mechanism of XZ-C immunomodulation of anticancer Chinese medicines is explained at the molecular level. It is very important.

1. XZ-C anti-cancer Chinese medicine can protect immune organs and enhance the quality of thymus and spleen.
2. XZ-C anticancer Chinese medicine has obvious promoting effect on bone marrow cell proliferation and hematopoietic function.
3. XZ-C anti-cancer Chinese medicine has an enhanced effect on T cell immune function, and has obvious promoting proliferation effect on T cells.
4. XZ-C anticancer Chinese medicine has a significant enhancement effect on the production of human 1L-2.
5. XZ-C5 anti-cancer Chinese medicine has a stimulating and potentiating effect on NK cells. NK cells have a broad-spectrum anti-tumor effect and can kill xenogenic tumor cells.
6. XZ-C anticancer Chinese medicine has an enhanced effect on the activity of LAK cells. LAK cells have a broad-spectrum anti-tumor effect on solid tumor cells that are sensitive to and sensitive to NK cells.
7. XZ-C anticancer Chinese medicine has the function of promoting tumor necrosis factor (TNF). TNF is a kind of cytokine which can directly cause tumor cell death. Its main biological function is to kill or inhibit tumor cells.

Biological response modifier (BRM) and BRM-like Chinese medicine and tumor treatment

1. Biological response modifier (BRM) has opened up a new field of tumor biotherapy. At present, BRM is widely regarded in the medical profession as the fourth program of tumor treatment.

In 1982, Oldham founded the biological response modifier (BRM), or BRM theory. On this basis, in 1984, he proposed the fourth modality of cancer treatment, biotherapy. According to the BRM theory, under normal circumstances, the dynamic balance between tumor and body defense, tumor occurrence and even invasion and metastasis are completely caused by the imbalance of this dynamic balance. If the state of the disorder has been artificially adjusted to a normal level, the growth of the tumor can be controlled and allowed to subside.

Specifically, BRM includes the following anti-tumor mechanisms:

1. to promote the enhancement of the effect of the host defense mechanism, or to reduce the immunosuppression of the tumor-bearing host, in order to achieve the immune response to cancer.
2. The natural or genetically recombinant biologically active substance is administered to enhance the defense mechanism of the host.
3. Modification of tumor cells induces a strong host response.
4. Promote the differentiation and maturation of tumor cells and normalize them.
5. to alleviate the toxic side effects of cancer chemotherapy and radiotherapy, and enhance the tolerance of the host.

2, BRM-like effect and efficacy of XZ-C immunomodulation of anti-cancer Chinese medicine

XZ-C immunomodulation anti-cancer Chinese medicine after 4 years of experimental research on cancer-bearing animals and 10 years of clinical verification showed that it has BRM-like effect and efficacy, and is a drug with BRM-like effect excavated from Chinese medicine resources. XZ-C immunomodulation anticancer Chinese medicine was experimentally screened from 200 Chinese herbal medicines by Professor Xu Ze's laboratory. Firstly, the cancer cells were cultured in vitro, and 200 kinds of Chinese herbal medicines were screened in vitro to observe the direct damage of the cancer cells in the culture tube, and the tumor cells were treated with the chemotherapy drug CTX and the normal cells in the test tube. Rate comparison test. As a result, a batch of drugs that have a certain cancer suppressing rate against cancer cell proliferation were selected. Then, the tumor-bearing animal model was further made, and the experimental study on the in vivo anti-tumor rate screening of the tumor-bearing animal model was carried out on 200 kinds of Chinese herbal medicines. The scientific, objective and rigorous experimental screening, analysis and evaluation were carried out. The results showed that only 48 species had a good tumor inhibition rate, and another 152 commonly used Chinese herbal medicines were screened by the tumor inhibition rate in this group of tumor-bearing experimental tumors, which showed no anticancer effect or a small tumor inhibition rate.

The XZ-C immunomodulatory anti-cancer metastasis drug that has been screened by the above experiments has improved immunity, increased thymus weight, protected thymus tissue function, increased cellular immunity, promoted bone marrow cell proliferation, and protected bone marrow blood production. Increase the number of red blood cells and white blood cells, enhance T cell function, activate immune cytokines, and improve immune surveillance in blood flow.

The main pharmacological action of XZ-C immunomodulation anticancer Chinese medicine is anti-cancer elevation, and its anti-cancer mechanism is:

1. Activate the body's immune cell system, promote the enhancement of the host defense mechanism, and achieve the immune response to cancer.
2. Activate the immune cytokine system of the body's anti-cancer mechanism, enhance the host defense mechanism and improve the immune surveillance of the immune cells of the body's blood circulation system.
3. protecting Thymus and increasing immune function, protect the thymus, increase immunity, protect the marrow from blood, protect the bone marrow from blood function, stimulate bone marrow hematopoietic function, promote the recovery of bone marrow suppression, increase white blood cells, red blood cells, etc.
4. to alleviate the side effects of radiotherapy and chemotherapy, and enhance the tolerance of the host.
5. it can increase the weight of the thymus, so that the thymus does not progressive atrophy, as the cancer progresses, the chest and chest progressive atrophy.

As mentioned above, the mechanism of action of XZ-C immunomodulatory anticancer Chinese medicine is basically similar to that of BRM, and the clinical use also obtains the same therapeutic effect of BRM. Therefore, XZ-C immunomodulation anticancer Chinese medicine has BRM-like effect and efficacy and combines today's advanced molecular oncology theory with ancient Chinese herbal medicine resources at the molecular level, Western medicine, BRM theory as a bridge, and the international advanced sub-oncology advanced theory and practice.

3, XZ-C1 + XZ-C4 immune regulation anti-cancer traditional Chinese medicine XZ-C1 + XZ-C4 immune regulation anti-cancer Chinese medicine has the following characteristics.

(1) Comprehensively improve the quality of life of patients with advanced cancer.
(2) Protect the thymus to improve immunity, protect bone marrow, enhance hematopoietic function, and improve immunity and regulation.
(3) Enhance physical fitness, reduce pain and increase appetite.
(4) Enhance the therapeutic effect and reduce the adverse reactions of chemotherapy.

6. XZ-C immunomodulation anticancer Chinese medicine is the result of modernization of traditional Chinese medicine

XZ-C immunomodulation anticancer traditional Chinese medicine is not an empirical method, nor is it an old Chinese medicine practitioner, but a scientific research achievement of the combination of Chinese and Western medicine and traditional Chinese medicine. It is a modern medical method, using experimental tumor research methods and modern pharmacology and medicine. Combining the effects of research methods, after more than 4,000 tumor-bearing animal models in 7 years, 200 commonly used anti-cancer Chinese herbal medicines were recorded in the literature, and screened in animal experiments in batches. The screening of tumor inhibition rates in vitro and in tumor-bearing animals was carried out one by one. 48 kinds of traditional Chinese medicines with good anti-cancer effects were screened out.

XZ-C immunomodulation Chinese medicine preparation is an innovation and reform of traditional Chinese medicine preparation. It is not a compound preparation for mixed decoction, but a particle concentrate or powder for each medicine. The raw material of each medicine still retains its original ingredients and pharmacology. The function, molecular weight and structural formula are unchanged, and are made by modern scientific methods, rather than compounding, keeping the original ingredients and functions of each flavor unchanged, and it is easy to evaluate and affirm the effects and effects of various medicines.

In the above series of studies, we spent 4 years exploring the mechanism and regularity of cancer metastasis, looking for an effective method for anti-cancer metastasis; and spent 3 years passing 200 scientifically controlled cancer-bearing animal models from 200 traditional anti-cancer Chinese herbal medicines. Screening of tumor inhibition rate, 48 kinds of XZ-C immunomodulatory anti-cancer and anti-metastatic traditional Chinese medicines with good tumor inhibition rate were screened out. Based on this experimental study, it has been applied to more than 10,000 patients with advanced cancer in the past 20 years, and has achieved good results. **From clinical to experimental, from experimental to clinical, the implementation of basic and clinical integration, the combination of Chinese and Western medicine at the molecular level, it intends to embark on a new road of anti-cancer and anti-metastasis with Chinese characteristics.** .

7, take XZ-C immune regulation, molecular level, Western medicine combined with the road to overcome cancer

The combination of Chinese and Western medicine is the characteristics and advantages of Chinese medicine. The goal of combining Chinese and Western medicine should be to combine innovation, and the goal of innovation should be to improve the treatment effect. The efficacy criteria for cancer patients should be: **long survival time, good quality of life, and few complications**.

Adhere to the direction of innovation between Chinese and Western medicine, and we should persevere.

Mr. Lu Xun once said that there is no road in the world, and many people are leaving the road. In the past 60 years, we have initially embarked on a new way to use immunomodulation of Chinese medicine, regulate immune activity, prevent thymic atrophy, promote thymic hyperplasia, protect bone marrow hematopoietic function, improve immune surveillance, and combine Western medicine at the molecular level to overcome cancer.

Achieving combined innovation and improving curative effect is the goal of combining high-level Chinese and Western medicine. It is necessary to combine not only traditional Chinese medicine theory with modern medical practice, but also to use experimental research to clarify the internal meaning of TCM theory, modern molecular oncology Chinese medicine immunopharmacology... ... the internal theory of modern oncology theory, and then in the theoretical and clinical practice to develop and innovate, thereby improving the treatment effect and benefiting patients.

Our experimental surgical research institute is based on the research direction and main task of conquering cancer. It is a joint research project to tackle cancer. It is a combination of Chinese and Western medicine. It is a combination of Chinese and Western medicine at the molecular level. On the basis of animal experiments, And in the clinical practice of clinical practice to achieve the combination of Chinese and Western medicine, and then in the anti-cancer, anti-cancer transfer theory development, innovation:

——Traditional Chinese medicine believes that righteousness is not empty, evil spirits do not enter, and the rule or governance must be based on strengthening the foundation and attaching importance to righting. Western medicine believes that tumors are low in immune function, and must be "protected by Thymus and Increasing immune" to enhance immunity.

Chinese medicine emphasizes righting up, which is equivalent to the immunity of Western medicine. The two are in good agreement.

——Traditional Chinese medicine cures not only pay attention to the righteousness but also to remove the evil spirits, that is, righting up strengthening the righteousness or to eliminate evil spirits. Western medicine believes that boosting immunity and improving immune surveillance, thus eliminating cancer cells on the way of metastasis, both of the treatment concepts are similar or the two are very consistent.

——Traditional Chinese medicine treatment of promoting the circulation and removing blood stasis is a common principle. In our research on anti-cancer metastasis, we realized that it is necessary to block cancer cells on the way of metastasis, anti-cancer, anticoagulation, anti-blood stasis, and promotion of blood circulation, improve blood rheology, and cure blood circulation in Chinese medicine. The rule of treatment is consistent with the rule of Western medicine for the treatment of cancer and metastasis.

Adhering to the scientific research work of combining Chinese and Western medicine with innovation, we should persevere and persevere, adhere to the road of independent innovation with

Chinese characteristics, and promote the new development of the theory of modern oncology in the 21st century.

Take the road of modernization of traditional Chinese medicine, promote the integration of Chinese and Western medicine at the molecular level, and integrate with the modernization of international medicine, and strive to take the road of innovation in anti-cancer and anti-cancer transformation with distinctive characteristics in China.

Now it is the second 10 years of the 21st century. It should be the era of innovation between Chinese and Western medicine. For more than 20 years, we have been focusing on improving the clinical efficacy of cancer as a major disease. Perseverance and perseverance, the monograph of the thesis (the third monograph "New Concepts and New Methods for Cancer Treatment" has been translated into English by American Dr. Bin Wu, and the English version has been published internationally) has been published. To study the theory of anti-cancer, anti-cancer metastasis and recurrence, develop a new modern anti-cancer, anti-metastatic traditional Chinese medicine preparation, XZ-C immune regulation anti-cancer traditional Chinese medicine preparation series (XZ-C1-10), the experimental research, basic research and clinical combination, medical and drug combination were carried out. The ancient Chinese herbal medicine was combined with traditional Chinese medicine immunology, molecular biology and cytokine science, complementing Chinese and Western, and combining innovation.

Efforts will be made to take the road of innovation in China's distinctive anti-cancer transfer, take the road of modernization of traditional Chinese medicine, promote the integration of Chinese and Western medicine at the molecular level, and integrate with international medicine modernization. We have initially embarked on a road of XZ-C immune regulation, molecular and Chinese medicine combined with cancer.

Printed in the United States
By Bookmasters